POISONING
EMERGENCIES
A PRIMER

Robert W. Jaeger, BS Pharm.
Operations Director, Cardinal Glennon Children's Hospital
Regional Poison Center
St. Louis, Missouri

and
Consultant
Fernando J. deCastro, MD, MPH
Clinical Professor, St. Louis University School of Medicine
Medical Director, Cardinal Glennon Children's Hospital
Regional Poison Center
St. Louis, Missouri

The Catholic Health Association of the United States
St. Louis, MO

Toxicology is a dynamic, ever progressive science. Doses of medication and procedures may change based on new information and case studies. The author of this primer has tried to assure that the doses of drugs are correct and are within generally accepted standards of use at the time of publication. However, the reader is cautioned to consult the manufacturer's and individual institution's procedure references regarding each drug or therapeutic agent prior to administration.

Library of Congress Cataloging-in-Publication Data

Jaeger, Robert W.
  Poisoning emergencies.

  Includes bibliographies and index.
  1. Poisoning, Accidental. 2. Poisons — Safety measures. I. Catholic Health Association of the United States. II. Title. [DNLM: 1. Emergencies. 2. Poisoning. 3. Poisons. QV 600 J22p]
  RA1224.5.J34 1987 615.9'08   86-29895
  ISBN 0-87125-123-X

Copyright©1987
by
The Catholic Health Association of the United States
4455 Woodson Road
St. Louis, MO 63134

Printed in the United States of America. All rights reserved. No part of this publication may be reproduced, stored in a retrieval system, or transmitted, in any form or by any means, electronic, mechanical, photocopying, recording, or otherwise, without the prior written permission of the publisher.

TABLE OF CONTENTS

INTRODUCTION

With approximately 5 million poisonings and 12,000 related fatalities occurring annually in the United States, the modern health care practitioner requires a working knowledge of the toxicity of common drugs and chemicals. The information presented in this manual will assist health care professionals in developing the knowledge and confidence necessary to effectively treat poisoned or overdosed patients.

This manual is organized into six major parts: Basic concepts, Chapters 1 to 4; drug poisoning and overdose, Chapters 5 to 13; household poisons, Chapters 14 to 19; industrial and occupational poisoning, Chapters 20 to 22; legal aspects, Chapter 23; and a guide to working in conjunction with a regional poison center, Chapter 24.

The manual is designed as a primer for the emergency care clinician and for students in medicine, nursing, and pharmacy. Registered nurses, licensed practical nurses, and technicians in accelerated programs will find the primer useful and comprehensive, as will industrial, occupational health, and school nurses. Paramedical police and firefighters can apply parts of the manual, particularly the sections on industrial toxicology, to their day-to-day work in the field.

The more dangerous drugs and chemicals are generally discussed in more detail under the Treatment subhead, which follows a discussion of each substance. Tables are used where appropriate to assist the reader in determining how soon a patient might have symptoms following an overdose or poisoning. Such knowledge is important when deciding what method of gastrointestinal decontamination to employ.

The index categorizes drug and chemical entries by both generic and brand name, as they occur in the text. Important terms are shown in boldface in the index.

In all, the book is intended to present material in a straightforward manner. The chapters on drugs and chemicals are more devoted to practical treatment than to theoretical pharmacology and toxicology. Although theory is discussed when necessary to clarify the rationale for treatment, attention is generally paid to alerting the clinician to expected signs and symptoms of overdose and conventional thinking with regard to medical management. Numerous excellent publications are devoted to theoretical pharmacology and toxicology, and they are suggested as additional readings in the Bibliography.

BASIC CONCEPTS

Chapters 1 through 4 present concepts that are basic to an understanding of the subject of clinical toxicology. Who gets poisoned? How does poisoning occur? What basic treatment is standard for all patients? What antidotes are currently recommended? How does the absorption, distribution, biotransformation, and excretion of drugs and chemicals affect the intensity of a toxic reaction? How does the clinical laboratory assist in the diagnosis of the poisoned patient? These subjects will be discussed in this first section.

This portion of the primer probably deals with more theoretical concepts than any other section. Although some of the pharmacokinetic concepts presented in Chapter 3 may be difficult to understand, every attempt has been made to simplify concepts that might be referred to in later chapters, particularly where knowledge of a theory is helpful in understanding a rationale for treatment.

CHAPTER 1 *GENERAL CONSIDERATIONS*

INCIDENCE

Historically, reports in the literature of the incidence rate for poisoning have ranged from a low of 1.5 per 1,000 to a high of 30 per 1,000 in the general population. The most recent data from the American Association of Poison Control Centers' National Data Collection System (representing the largest poison exposure database ever compiled in the United States) show that reports of exposures from participating poison centers range from 2.1 to 20.2 per 1,000 with a mean of 7.9 reported exposures per 1,000. These data, when extrapolated to the population of the United States, predict a nationwide annual incidence of human poison exposures over 1.9 million. The National Data Collection System uses what it calls "poison center penetrance" (defined as the number of human poison exposure cases reported to a center divided by the population served by the center) to explain these reported rates, a concept somewhat analogous to "market saturation" in a given region, since to a large extent the number of cases reported to a poison center depends on how well known the service is in the region. Therefore, assuming all centers in the United States reached the maximum "penetrance" level of 20.2 exposures per 1,000 population, then almost 5 million poisonings would be reported annually. Of course, it is difficult to extrapolate the number of actual poisonings (patients with symptoms) from the frequency of reported poisonings, but it is apparent from these figures that the extent of human morbidity, economic burden, and expenditure of medical services is enormous. Also, the number of deaths reported to poison centers annually is an underestimate of the national problem, since many exposures that are discovered too late for treatment are never brought to the attention of a poison center. Thus the resulting 12,000 fatalities that are reported annually by the Food and Drug Administration's Poisoning Surveillance and Epidemiology Branch (formerly the National Clearing House for Poison Control Centers) are collected from Poison Centers, the National Institute on Drug Abuse's Drug Abuse Warning Network (DAWN), and the National Center for Health Statistics mortality data. Not only does this figure not include envenomations, late effects of poisoning, carbon monoxide deaths from fires, medical complications and misadventures such as adverse drug reactions and anesthetic overdoses, and various conditions such as pneumoconioses resulting from chronic exposure to toxic materials, but it is an underestimate of the actual number of deaths due to toxic substances following accidental exposure in children and adults, drug abuse-related deaths, and suicide in older children and adults.

DEMOGRAPHICS

Children ingest poisons accidentally more often in the 1- to 5- year age group, with a peak at 18 months of age. Children under 6 years of age constitute about 65 percent of all exposures reported to poison centers in the United States. The great majority of poisonings reported to poison centers are accidental. According to reporting centers, a slight male predominance is seen in victims under 13 years of age, but the gender distribution is reversed in teenagers and adults. Although accidental poisonings seem to outnumber both intentional poisonings and adverse reactions in all age groups, the ratio is lower in teenager and adult cases, with suicidal gestures and drug abuse attempts accounting for the shift. The most common time of the day in which toxic exposures occur is the late afternoon and early evening, between 5:00 and 8:00 PM. The late morning is the next most common time period; many of these exposures are accidental ingestions in toddlers. The time of day when ingestions occur most frequently suggests that children ingest toxic substances more often during family disorganization or disruption. The two peak times seem to correspond with times when the household is more chaotic. Also, when the status quo of the family is disturbed, such as by divorce, separation, death, or relocation, children tend to ingest toxic substances more often.

PREVENTION

Preventing accidental poisoning should be a major concern of health care professionals. More than two thirds of accidental poisonings in children occur from ingestion of compounds that are in household use. Several other factors, such as age, place, time of day, and family disruption, must be considered to prevent accidental poisoning. Remember that accidental poisoning is not only a problem of childhood. It frequently occurs among older persons who inadvertently receive or give household chemicals mistaken for medications, and it happens as a result of occupational exposure to noxious chemicals.

Suicide is a major psychiatric problem, particularly among adolescents, and frequently involves poisoning in addition to firearms and hanging as the means of death. Although poisoning accounts for only 25 percent of the fatalities due to suicide in persons under age 25, it is by far the most common mode of suicide *gesture*. Although the psychosocial issues of suicide are not within the scope of this book, the substances that are frequently involved in suicide attempts are discussed.

POISON PREVENTION PACKAGING

The Uniform Hazardous Substance Act (1960) requires a household toxic substance to be labeled with the word Warning, Caution, Danger, or Poison, depending on its toxicity. The newer Fair Packaging Labeling Act includes safety labeling for nonprescription drugs, medical devices, and cosmetics. More recently, the 1970 Poison Prevention Packaging Act, administered by the Consumer Product Safety Commission (CPSC), provides that certain household products that are found to be hazardous or potentially hazardous must be sold in safety packaging that most children under 5 years of age cannot open if these products are in packages for use in or around the household. Currently required to be in safety packaging by regulations promulgated under the Poison Prevention Packaging Act are the following drugs and chemicals:

1. Aspirin. Any aspirin-containing preparation for human use in a dosage form intended for oral administration, except some effervescent tablets and unflavored aspirin-containing preparations in powder form.

2. Furniture polish. Nonemulsion-type liquid furniture polishes containing 10 percent or more of mineral seal oil or other petroleum distillates and having a viscosity of less than 100 Saybolt universal seconds at 100°F, other than those packaged in pressurized spray containers.

3. Methyl salicylate. Liquid preparations containing more than 5 percent by weight of methyl salicylate, other than those packaged in pressurized spray containers.

4. Controlled drugs. Any preparation for human use that consists wholly or partially of any substance subject to control under the Comprehensive Drug Abuse Prevention and Control Act of 1970 and that is in a dosage form intended for oral administration.

5. Sodium or potassium hydroxide. Household substances in dry forms such as granules, powder, and flakes, containing 10 percent or more by weight of free or chemically unneutralized sodium or potassium hydroxide, and all other household substances containing 2 percent or

more by weight of free or chemically unneutralized sodium or potassium hydroxide.

6. Turpentine. Household substances in liquid form containing 10 percent or more by weight of turpentine.

7. Kindling or illuminating preparations. Prepackaged liquid kindling or illuminating preparations (cigarette lighter fuel, charcoal lighter fuel, camping equipment fuel, torch fuel, and fuel for decorative or functional lanterns) that contain 10 percent or more by weight of petroleum distillates and have a viscosity of less than 100 Saybolt universal seconds at 100°F.

8. Methyl alcohol (methanol). Household substances in liquid form containing 4 percent or more by weight of methyl alcohol (methanol), other than those packaged in pressurized spray containers.

9. Sulfuric acid. Household substances containing 10 percent or more by weight of sulfuric acid, except such substances in wet-cell storage batteries.

10. Prescription drugs. Any drug for human use that is in a dosage form intended for oral administration and that is required by federal law to be dispensed only by or on an oral or written prescription of a practitioner licensed by law, *except for the following:*

a. Sublingual dosage forms of nitroglycerin.

b. Sublingual and chewable forms of isosorbide dinitrate in dosage strengths of 10 mg or less.

c. Erythromycin ethylsuccinate granules for oral suspension in packages containing not more than 8 g of the equivalent of erythromycin.

d. Cyclically administered oral contraceptives in manufacturers' mnemonic (memory-aid) dispenser packages that rely solely on the activity of one or more progestogen or estrogen substances.

e. Anhydrous cholestyramine in powder form.

f. All unit dose forms of potassium supplements, including individually wrapped effervescent tablets, unit dose vials of liquid potassium, and powdered potassium in unit dose packets, containing not more than 50 mEq of potassium per unit dose.

g. Sodium fluoride drug preparations, including liquid and tablet forms, containing no more than 264 mg of sodium fluoride per package.

h. Betamethasone tablets packaged in manufacturers' dispenser packages, containing no more than 12.6 mg of betamethasone.

i. Pancrelipase preparations in tablet, capsule, or powder form.

j. Prednisone in tablet form when dispensed in packages containing no more than 105 mg of the drug.

k. Mebendazole in tablet form in packages containing not more than 600 mg of the drug.

l. Methylprednisolone in tablet form in packages containing not more than 84 mg of the drug.

m. Colestipol in powder form in packages containing not more than 5 g of the drug.

n. Erythromycin ethylsuccinate tablets in packages containing no more than the equivalent of 16 g of erythromycin.

o. Conjugated estrogen tablets, USP, when dispensed in mnemonic packages containing not more than 26.5 mg of the drug.

p. Norethindrone acetate tablets, USP, when dispensed in mnemonic packages containing not more than 50 mg of the drug.

11. Ethylene glycol. Household substances in liquid form containing 10 percent or more by weight of ethylene glycol packaged on or after June 1, 1974.

12. Iron-containing drugs, with some exceptions for animal feeds and unit dose packaging.

13. Dietary supplements containing iron, with the exception of those preparations in which iron is present solely as a colorant.

14. Solvents for paint or other similar surface coating material. Prepackaged liquid solvents (e.g., removers, thinners, brush cleaners) for paints or other similar surface coating materials (e.g., varnishes and lacquers) that contain 10 percent or more by weight of benzene (also known as benzol), toluene (also known as toluol), xylene (also known as xylol), petroleum distillates (e.g., gasoline, kerosene, mineral seal oil, mineral spirits, naphtha, and Stoddard solvents) or combinations thereof and that have a viscosity of less than 100 Saybolt universal seconds at 100°F.

15. Acetaminophen. Preparations for human use in a dosage form intended for oral administration and containing in a single package a total of more than 1 g of acetaminophen, except effervescent and unflavored, powdered products.

16. Diphenhydramine. Preparations for human use in a dosage form intended for oral administration and containing more than the equivalent of 66 mg of diphenhydramine base in a single package.

The child-resistant containers for these substances must be sufficiently difficult so that they cannot be opened by 80 percent of children under 5, but they must allow access to at least 90 percent of adults, who will then be able to open and properly close the packaging conveniently.

Exemptions have been granted for drugs to which patients need rapid access. These are mentioned above under no. 10, Prescription Drugs. Other drugs have been proposed for exemption. Future regulations will cover veterinary prescription drugs. For those few people, the very old and those with handicaps such as arthritis, who may find it impossible to use this new safety packaging, the law allows two ways to provide the traditional, easy-to-open packaging:

1. A manufacturer can market one size of the product in conventional packaging if other packages of the same product are on the market in safety packaging. However, in these exceptions, the label must clearly state: "This package for households without young children." Or, if the package is small: "Package not child resistant."

2. The prescribing physician or consumer may request that prescription medicines be put into ordinary packaging without safety features. Although some pharmacists may ask for a written statement from a purchaser before providing a conventional closure, this is not required by federal law.

Safety closures when used properly have demonstrated their effectiveness since 1972. Although the most recent data from poison centers clearly indicate that there is no decline in the number of incidents occurring each year, there is certainly a reduction in poison morbidity and mortality since implementation of the Poison Prevention Packaging Act. However, many circumstances exist in which one may be exposed to potentially poisonous chemicals and drugs, and, there is no reason to expect a decline in poisoning frequency because of many other problem areas, namely, suicide, drug abuse, occupational accidents including eye injuries from chemicals, skin contamination and inhalation, envenomations, environmental pollutants, and chemicals spills.

References — Chapter 1

D. J., Brancato, and R. C. Nelson, "Poisoning Mortality in the United States." *Vet. Hum. Tox.* 26:273-275, 1984.

Code of Federal Regulations, Title 16(16CFR), Chapter II 1700.14, January 1985 (substances requiring special packaging).

T. Litovitz, and J. C. Veltri, "1985 Annual Report of the American Association of Poison Control Centers National Data Collection System." *Am. J. Emerg. Med.* 4:427-458, 1986.

M. S. McIntire, and C. R. Angle, *Suicide Attempts in Children and Youth.* (Hagerstown, MD: Harper & Row, 1980).

D. K. Olson, et al., "An Epidemiological View of Poisoning." *Vet. Hum. Tox.* 27:402-408, 1985.

CHAPTER 2 *EMERGENCY TREATMENT*

Accidental and suicidal poisonings have been medical problems for generations but traditionally have received little attention. In the past 30 years, however, the problem of poisoning, particularly in industrialized nations, has received more emphasis. In the developed countries reduced childhood mortality from infectious diseases as a result of immunization and the introduction of specific antimicrobial therapy since the late 1940s have allowed physicians to recognize the magnitude of the medical problems caused by accidental poisoning. Since the early 1950s various organizations have been formed in different countries to deal more effectively with accidental poisoning. In the United States, a subcommittee on accidental poisoning was formed by the American Academy of Pediatrics, the American Association of Poison Control Centers, and more recently the American Academy of Clinical Toxicology. In Europe, as early as 1949 a specialized ward for clinical toxicology was functioning in Budapest, Hungary, and at about the same time an information service was set up in a hospital in Leeds, England. Subsequently, numerous effective services for poison control have been developed in Europe, such as the Gaullier Emergency Service in Paris and the National Poison Information Service in England.

This chapter is limited to one particular aspect of poisoning, that of emergency management. Although from the public health standpoint *preventing* poisoning is vital, emergency management is essential to the health care professional called to treat a patient after the poisoning episode has occurred. In fact, adequate emergency management can often be lifesaving. The differential diagnosis of a comatose patient should always include convulsion, infection, trauma, tumor, metabolic disorder, and poisoning.

To handle patients after a poisoning incident has occurred, the clinician must be able to identify the poisoning agent promptly to develop a rational therapy, not only in removing the toxic product but also in administering specific pharmacologic antagonists, in aiding excretion, and even in establishing rational supportive therapy. Access to identifying resources is crucial in this first step of emergency management. Poison centers are a resource for this type of information and assist the clinician in identification and diagnosis.

POISONING BY INGESTION

Ingestion is the most common route of poisoning. Once a toxic agent has been ingested, the clinician must be concerned with two aspects: (1) eliminating it from the patient's gastrointestinal tract to prevent absorption and (2) diminishing the effective dose absorbed.

Elimination from the Gastrointestinal Tract

In a sense, chemicals and drugs in the gastrointestinal tract are still outside the body because they have not yet become available to the bloodstream and target organs. Thus, steps must be taken to dilute the toxic substance, delay or prevent its absorption, or evacuate the gastrointestinal tract. In a few selected cases, the poison might be altered to produce a less toxic or inert product, such as when oral phosphate salts are administered to a person who has ingested ferrous sulfate, producing an inert iron-phosphate complex.

Dilution. To dilute an ingested poison, water or milk not exceeding 5 ml/kg body weight can be given. If the above amount is exceeded, gastric content can be forced past the pylorus and absorption enhanced, or if irritants are involved and emesis is contraindicated, vomiting might be induced. Milk may be used as a diluting agent because its protein and fat content enable it to act as a demulcent. This may be particularly helpful following the ingestion of irritant substances such as acids or alkali. However, dilution is not routinely recommended for drug ingestions, since it may enhance dissolution and absorption of the dosage form. When emesis is indicated following an ingestion, oral fluids may also be given, up to a higher dose of approximately 15 ml/kg in children and up to 300 ml total in adults. Although recent studies question the need for fluids with forced induction of emesis, it seems logical that some volume of liquid must be present in the stomach to effect a forceful emesis. This will be discussed in more detail shortly.

Decreasing absorption. Activated carbon or charcoal is used to physically adsorb the poison on the surface of its particles. Activated charcoal, an odorless, tasteless, fine black powder, is the residue from the destructive distillation of various organic materials (e.g., wood pulp) suitably treated to increase its surface area and adsorptive capacity.

The efficacy of activated charcoal as an adsorptive agent for substances in the gastrointestinal tract has been shown in numerous studies with aspirin, barbiturates, chloroquine, chlorpheniramine, chlorpromazine, glutethimide, propoxyphene, sodium salicylate, strychnine, and other substances. The dose of activated charcoal has been estimated to be at least 10 times the estimated dose of the poison. For practical purposes a minimum dose of 30 g in adults and 15 g in children, in 8 and 4 oz of liquid, respectively, is sufficient as a beginning dose; however, doses up to 100 g can be given in adults when the drug and the quantity ingested are unknown. Activated charcoal is commercially available in several vehicles; water and 70 percent sorbitol are probably the two most commonly used. When sorbitol is used as a vehicle for charcoal, remember that it can cause spontaneous emesis and fluid deficit. Sorbitol is preferable in a patient who will drink the mixture, since sorbitol is a polyalcohol of sorbose that renders activated charcoal slurries sweet and thick. A cathartic is not necessary following sorbitol-based charcoal because sorbitol is an osmotic cathartic. If activated charcoal is administered through an orogastric or a nasogastric tube, use a water-based slurry to minimize irritation of the stomach and subsequent vomiting while the tube is inserted.

Evacuation. Evacuation of the gastrointestinal tract can be accomplished best by emesis or orogastric lavage and also by laxatives and enemas.

Do not attempt emesis by gagging, particularly in children. Although some clinicians feel there is a risk of tissue injury or penetration, particularly in small children, it simply is not an effective way to empty the stomach and delays effective treatment. It is always important to know when *not* to induce emesis. Emesis is contraindicated for caustic agents and may not be indicated for a few petroleum distillates, particularly the extremely volatile substances such as mineral seal oil, which is found in some furniture polishes. Emesis after ingestion of caustic agents (alkaline or acid) may cause esophageal perforation. Many petroleum distillates (particularly aliphatic hydrocarbons) are not absorbed from the gastrointestinal tract, and therefore emesis is unnecessary because no systemic effects will occur. However, when other agents, such as metals and pesticides, are carried in hydrocarbon solvents, it may then be appropriate to induce vomiting. Aspiration complications with hydrocarbons have been shown to be the result of coughing and choking during ingestion, not emesis. Whatever minor risk of aspiration that exists during emesis is certainly outweighed by the benefits of prompt emesis following ingestion of common solutes in hydrocarbon vehicles, such as selenium salts (gun bluing compounds) and concentrated organophosphate pesticides.

Emesis may also be recommended following the ingestion of hydrocarbons if the quantity ingested exceeds 1 ml/kg. This volume is large enough to usually only occur in intentional ingestions. With large quantities sufficient gastritis may occur to overide protective physiologic barriers to absorption. However, remember that quantities determined from histories are usually exaggerations. Aspiration pneumonia does not appear to occur more frequently in patients who have been made to vomit following hydrocarbon ingestion than in patients who vomit spontaneously. If aspiration pneumonia occurs, antibiotics may be used if secondary infection of the chemical pneumonia is present (see Chap. 15 on hydrocarbons). The use of corticosteroids is of no value.

Syrup of ipecac. Syrup of ipecac is the most commonly used emetic. The syrup is prepared from an extract obtained from the dried rhizome and root of two plant species, *Cephaelis ipecacuanha* and *Cephaelis acuminata*. Primarily two alkaloids, emetine and cephaeline, are known to be responsible for the emetic effect. These alkaloids are known to have a central effect of stimulating the chemoreceptor trigger zone to cause vomiting. A lesser but local irritant effect is exhibited on the gastric and esophageal mucosa. Syrup of ipecac remains available without a prescription in 1-oz bottles according to the U.S. Code of Federal Regulations (21 CFR 369.21, 1985). Since it is safe and easily available for induction of emesis at home, ipecac is the emetic of choice in poisoning or overdose. The effective dose and ritual administration of syrup of ipecac have been debated in the medical and toxicologic literature for the last 30 years. Although ipecac induces emesis in nearly 100 percent of patients, its effectiveness in emptying the stomach contents has been questioned. Studies have demonstrated that approximately one third of test materials (chemical markers) are returned by emesis following administration of syrup of ipecac, and this is in a clinical setting under controlled conditions. Additionally, case reports have occurred in the literature documenting major complications from a single dose of syrup of ipecac administered for the treatment of poisoning. These include diaphragmatic rupture and death in a child aged 2 years and aspiration pneumonitis. Activated charcoal is becoming increasingly important as an alternative to emesis, and this will be discussed shortly. Nonetheless, syrup of ipecac remains useful in many situations, and the following procedure for its use is based on the American Association of Poison Control Centers' Scientific Review Committee recommendations:

1. When indicated, syrup of ipecac may be given according to the following guidelines:

a. Children under 1 year of age: Syrup of ipecac should be administered only under adequate medical supervision, necessitating that most children be referred to an emergency care facility. Very young infants may not be able to control head and neck muscles adequately and thus may be unable to protect against aspiration of vomitus. For children 6 months to under 1 year of age, 1 to 2 teaspoonfuls (5 to 10 ml) may be given in a controlled setting if necessary.

b. Children between the ages of 1 and 12 years: 1 table-spoonful (15 ml). Although some regional poison centers have begun to recommend 30 ml of ipecac in this age range, it is difficult to determine at what age to administer the adult dose. The American Association of Poison Control Centers does not believe that the scientific literature provides enough evidence to support the requirement to use only the 30-ml dose. Individual studies have been equivocal. In adults, studies indicate onset of emesis and percent effectiveness to be similar at 15 and 30 ml. In children, some research undertaken by regional poison centers indicates more rapid onset with 30 ml, but these studies are based on telephone history and retrospective follow-up studies rather than on on-site clinical evaluation.

c. Adults and children over 12 years of age: 1 to 2 table-spoonfuls (15 to 30 ml).

2. Administer fluids to fill the stomach adequately: children, 15 ml/kg; adults, up to 300 ml.

3. If emesis has not occurred within 20 minutes, repeat the dose of ipecac.

Cautions regarding ipecac and emesis — Ipecac was recognized as an effective emetic over 100 years ago, and the fact that it is used so extensively today in thousands of children each year attests to a reasonable safety record. However, as with any drug, it has limitations, precautions, side-effects, and adverse reactions that must be discussed. As previously mentioned, only one third to half of gastric contents may be recovered following ipecac-induced emesis. Therefore, do not rely on it as the only method of evacuating the gastrointestinal tract, particularly in serious or life-threatening overdoses. Ipecac is believed to be cardiotoxic in high enough doses, although one report states that one child retained 105 ml of the syrup with no effects. However, never use ipecac in concentrated preparations, such as the powdered extract or fluid extract (these preparations are no longer available at the retail level).

Do not induce emesis following the ingestion of corrosive chemicals, acids, and alkalies; on emesis, these materials may burn the soft tissues of the esophagus, pharynx, and mouth a second time. Induce emesis cautiously when central nervous system depressants have been ingested, since the patient must remain able to protect his airway. Emesis is contraindicated if the patient is comatose or has ingested certain convulsant chemicals, particularly camphor and strychnine. If the patient is comatose, aspiration may follow; and if a convulsant has been ingested, emesis may precipitate seizures. In these instances, activated charcoal,in water alone, is indicated.

After emesis has been accomplished, have the patient take nothing by mouth for the next 1½ to 2 hours. This allows the central effects of the alkaloids of ipecac to be cleared. If food and fluids are continued during this time, protracted vomiting may develop and lead to complications. Emesis occurring beyond the 2-hour observation period may be due to the ingested substance rather than to the syrup of ipecac, although an occasional child may be more sensitive to the gastric irritant effects of ipecac. In any case, observe children in particular very closely within this time period.

Following emesis children frequently become drowsy. If the drowsiness is attributable to emesis and not to ingestion, that is, if drowsiness is not an expected symptom of the substance ingested, it may be acceptable to allow the child to lie down or sleep. If the child lies down, keep him on his abdomen or side to preclude possible further episodes of emesis from resulting in aspiration. In any case, after completing the initial emesis at home or in an emergency facility, be aware of the possibility of further vomiting. Conscientious follow-up examination is critical to the successful administration of emetics and the patient's well-being, particularly when an ingestion is managed at home.

Alternatives of syrup of ipecac. Apomorphine hydrochloride, a parenterally administered drug, is used for its emetic effect. Apomorphine, a narcotic, is not as accessible as ipecac. It has the advantage over ipecac that it can be given parenterally and that its onset of action is usually faster than ipecac. However, it has serious disadvantages, since it is a narcotic analgesic and depresses respiration and the central nervous system. Apomorphine hydrochloride is administered subcutaneously in a dose of 0.1 mg/kg of body weight. Because of its possible respiratory depressant effect, administration of the narcotic antagonist naloxone hydrochloride is recommended after apomorphine-induced emesis. This means that a patient must receive numerous injections. In all, it is too difficult and too dangerous and can no longer be recommended for children.

The only safe alternative to syrup of ipecac as an emetic appears to be the use of certain anionic and nonionic detergents, the types used as dishwashing liquids, such as alkyl benzene sulfonates and sodium lauryl sulfate. Some protocols use 30 ml of detergent diluted in 240 ml (8 oz) of water or KoolAid to induce emesis. However, even though certain detergents are clearly safe when administered in controlled settings, there is always the danger of misunderstanding and possible confusion among laundry, dish, and electric dishwasher products. Some products may not induce emesis; others, containing alkaline "builders" and additional chemicals, may be corrosive. A detergent emetic may be judiciously used by regional poison centers but certainly is not generally advised for the public.

Gastric lavage. Gastric lavage by nasal or oral intubation has traditionally been used to evacuate the gastrointestinal tract. Emesis appears to be superior or equal to gastric lavage in emptying the stomach, but gastric lavage is unquestionably indicated in the treatment of poisoned patients who are in coma, are convulsing, or have no gag reflex. Furthermore, it facilitates the administration of activated charcoal. It may be quite difficult to have certain patients drink large doses of activated charcoal, but activated charcoal can be administered quite easily through a tube. As with emesis, gastric lavage is contraindicated if patients have ingested corrosive or caustic products.

Gastric lavage literally washes the stomach ("lavage" from the Latin *lavare*, to wash). Following poisoning, and particularly drug overdoses in adolescents and adults, normal gastric lavage with standard-size nasogastric tubes and lavage syringes is ineffective in emptying the stomach quickly and efficiently. Use a procedure employing a tube and funnel to instill and drain up to 20 liters of lavage fluid in and out of the stomach very quickly. Attach a funnel to the end of a no. 36 French or larger orogastric tube after inserting it into the patient's stomach. Fill the funnel with 100 to 200 ml of solution and raise it to allow filling of the stomach. Lower the tube and funnel into a container under or below the patient so that gastric emptying occurs by gravity. Take care to prevent aspiration of drippings during withdrawal of the tube from the patient.

Laxatives. Laxatives are not as effective as gastric lavage or emesis in removing ingested toxic products, but they are useful, since rapid catharsis is also important to remove unabsorbed material from the intestine. Take care in determining the potential value of the laxative for a specific ingested substance, since laxatives themselves may induce problems due to absorption of cations. Magnesium sulfate (Epsom salt), sodium sulfate (Glauber salt), sodium phosphate (Fleet's phosphosoda), and citrate of magnesia (magnesium citrate solution) are all relatively safe cathartics for use in poisoning. Keep in mind that saline cathartics such as sodium sulfate or phosphate may induce hypernatremia. Some oil-based cathartics may be useful following certain types of drug and chemical ingestions because of their ligand-forming properties that result in complexes in the gastrointestinal tract. However, castor oil and mineral oil may be hazardous if aspirated, causing a lipoid pneumonia.

Enemas. Enemas are also of value in reducing the absorption of toxic substances from the gastrointestinal tract. However, their value in eliminating ingested toxic substances is much more limited.

Diminishing the Effective Dose

The first step in handling ingestion is to eliminate the ingested poison from the gastrointestinal tract. However, since the elimination procedures are not usually fully effective, the physican must also take steps towards diminishing the effective dose of the ingested absorbed poison. Some such steps are administering antidotes, facilitating excretion in the urine, and performing other therapeutic interventions, such as peritoneal dialysis, renal dialysis, charcoal hemoperfusion, and exchange transfusion.

Pharmacologic antagonists. Specific "antidotes" or pharmacologic antagonists for toxic substances are relatively few, but when they exist, they are of definite value in the management of the poisoned patient. For example, atropine can be administered to patients intoxicated by organophosphate insecticides, which are cholinesterase inhibitors; and for patients poisoned with a narcotic analgesic, such as methadone, naloxone hydrochloride is of value. Other antagonists are discussed later in this chapter.

Forced diuresis. Elimination of a toxic substance can also be achieved by forced diuresis, since numerous substances are excreted in the urine. In such instances, increasing urinary flow by giving large quantities of oral, rectal, or, more dependably, intravenous fluid will help eliminate the toxic substance faster in the glomerular filtrate. Forced diuresis is even more effective if the pH of the urine is adjusted with appropriate intravenous therapy, such as in aspirin toxicity when an alkaline urine helps eliminate larger quantities of the drug. In aspirin toxicity alkalinization of the urine has been successfully tried with the administration of either sodium bicarbonate intravenously or the carbonic anhydrase inhibitor acetazolamide. Phenobarbital is also eliminated faster in an alkaline urine. On the other hand, amphetamines and phencyclidine are eliminated better in an acid urine.

Dialysis and exchange transfusion. Dialysis may be lifesaving in patients who have ingested very large doses of water-soluble poisons such as aspirin, heavy metals in conjunction with chelation, some barbiturates and very toxic water-soluble substances such as methanol, and ethylene glycol. Exchange transfusion is another heroic procedure of more limited value than are peritoneal and renal dialysis. Exchange transfusion can be of help in treating poisoning from the same substances dialysis addresses and also in poisoning from some agents that are plasma protein bound (e.g., iron) or blood element bound (e.g., production of methemoglobinemia). Exchange transfusion and dialysis can be lifesaving but often do not offer a great advantage over the more conservative treatment of forced diuresis with proper adjustment of the urinary pH, and they certainly carry a much greater morbidity.

Dialysis is contraindicated in patients intoxicated with substances that are fat soluble or protein or tissue bound, such as tricyclic antidepressants, antihistamines, benzodiazepines, narcotic analgesics, phenothiazine tranquilizers, and glutethimide. Lipid dialysis is a new technique that is of value in patients who have ingested previously nondializable substances such as tranquilizers and glutethimide.

POISONING BY SKIN CONTAMINATION

Toxic chemicals may produce pathologic effects when they come in contact with the skin. These agents may not only produce surface damage, but also may induce pathophysiologic changes due to systemic absorption through the skin. Skin contact is the most important route of exposure in industrial toxicity.

When the surface of the skin is exposed to a toxic chemical, promptly irrigate the area with copious amounts of water or any other available liquid. Preferably, place the involved area under a stream of water for a minimum of 15 minutes, washing it thoroughly with soap and water. After irrigation, neutralization of strong bases or acids is sometimes desirable. For example, vinegar, which is a weak acid, and bicarbonate of soda, which is a weak base, can be used but are of limited value. Neutralizing agents are often unavailable. Furthermore, an unexpected event may occur such as more damage derived from the heat of an exothermic reaction if irrigation is not thorough.

Chemicals may not only damage the skin but may produce systemic toxicity by absorption through the skin, as in chlorinated and organophosphate insecticides. Once skin exposure occurs, promptly wash the involved area with soap and water and treat the systemic effect as described in the preceding section (absorbed ingested poisons).

POISONING BY INHALATION

Patients may also be poisoned by inhalation, and as with skin contamination, the damage may be due to local irritation of the respiratory tract or to systemic absorption.

Immediately carry the poisoned patient to fresh air and loosen the clothing. When patients' respiration is depressed, mouth-to-mouth resuscitation (CPR) or even intratracheal intubation and intermittent positive pressure breathing with oxygen may be necessary. Since a prolonged expiratory phase during artificial ventilation will impair return of venous blood, pressure must be monitored. If needed, conserve body heat by applying blankets. Use specific antidotes, if available, for those inhaled toxic products producing systemic toxicity, such as amyl nitrite for cyanide poisoning.

EYE CONTAMINATION

When eye contamination occurs, the importance of time so outweighs other considerations that tap water or the first innocuous watery solution at hand should be used to irrigate the eye. Continuous irrigation of the conjunctival sac can be accomplished using intravenous fluids (normal saline) after a topical anesthetic has been administered in the emergency room. In chemical burns of the eye it has been suggested that cooler liquids at the beginning may help reduce the heat of some chemical reactions, but this has not been experimentally validated.

Since many substances do not bind chemically with tissues and are readily water soluble and eliminated by irrigation, prompt brief irrigation (about 3 to 5 minutes) usually should suffice.

Prolonged irrigation (20 to 30 minutes) is necessary immediately after initial contamination of the eye with strong alkalies, since in these cases the pH of the conjunctival sac may take minutes to return to the normal range. Test the conjunctival sac with wide-range pH test paper every 5 to 10 minutes in the course of irrigation to measure the rate at which the pH is returning to a tolerable value such as 8 or 8.5. Do not expect a pH of 7. In acid burns the pH of the conjunctival sac may return to normal range during irrigation more quickly than in alkali burns. As far as is known, nothing is gained by continued irrigation after the pH has definitely returned to normal. Extended irrigation is also recommended for other chemically reactive substances or those with an oily or viscous base (e.g., hydrocarbons). When the nature of the substance is unknown, irrigate excessively rather than inadequately to be safe.

If there is any possibility of contamination with solid particles, it is vital to search the conjunctival sac. Completely evert the lids and remove the particles mechanically as quickly as possible, continuing irrigation while doing so. A drop of local anesthetic can make this procedure easier and more comfortable for the patient.

Fluorescein may be used to uncover epithelial damage on the cornea or the conjunctiva. Remember that tests with fluorescein cannot be depended on to rule out injury in all cases, since symptoms of damage can be latent, sometimes for several hours after exposure. Latent periods of this sort are most commonly encountered after exposure to gases, vapors, and fumes but can also occur after contact with certain liquids and solids (e.g., ethylene oxide, hydrogen sulfides, or sodium hypochlorite-ammonia mixtures). The slit-lamp microscope and ophthalmoscope can be relied on for more detailed information in all cases of eye contamination.

Although neutralizing chemical contaminants with various reagents has been proposed, and despite its theoretical advantage (neutralized alkalies with acids and vice versa), this type of neutralization has seldom been shown to provide a significant improvement over immediate irrigation with water or saline (which is usually much more readily available for first-aid treatment). There are a few instances in which specific antidotes are advantageous. (See Chap. 22 for a more extensive discussion on eye contamination.)

SUPPORTIVE THERAPY

Establishing an adequate airway and cardiopulmonary resuscitation; maintaining body temperature, nutrition status, and fluid and electrolyte balance; and preventing or promptly treating circulatory collapse, hypoglycemia, uremia, and liver failure are all well-known aspects of supportive therapy to maintain vital functions during the critical periods when the poison may overwhelm the patient.

Frequently in cases of poisoning the only therapy available is supportive therapy. If adequately administered, supportive care may lead to recovery more often than more dramatic or even heroic treatment. Supportive therapy if properly administered maintains life and allows restorative processes to overcome the pathophysiologic aberration induced by the poison. Nonetheless, a few certain "antidotes" do exist and may also be lifesaving when indicated in poisoning. These are discussed in the following section.

PHARMACOLOGIC AGENTS USED IN THE MANAGEMENT OF THE POISONED PATIENT

Specific pharmacologic antagonists that may be used for poisoning are discussed below. At one time the term *antidote*, which literally means to be "given against," was employed to describe these substances. However, it has become clear in modern times that few poisons have such well-understood and defined physiologic mechanisms that one specific agent can be used as an "antidote" to antagonize its activity. The grouping below is helpful in thinking of drugs and chemicals in terms of their usefulness in poisoning:

1. Pharmacologic antagonists
2. Chelating agents
3. Supportive drugs
4. Emetics, absorbents, and cathartics
5. Antivenins and biologicals
6. "Ion-trapping" drugs

The following, although not all-inclusive, is intended to present the most commonly employed drugs and techniques in the management of the poisoned-overdosed patient.

Pharmacologic Antagonists (closest to the classic concept of "antidote")

Atropine sulfate injection — a cholinergic blocking agent effective in the treatment of poisoning from anticholinesterase agents. It is also occasionally used in the treatment of drug-induced bradycardia. A test dose of 2 mg intravenously is standard in adults. In children, 0.05 mg/kg intravenously up to 2 mg may be used. The end point of treatment is to keep the patient dry, i.e., cessation of secretions, not just dilatation of pupils. Since atropine is used to antagonize acetylcholine, as much as 2 g daily has been used to keep patients only mildly atropinized.

Cyanide antidote kit — management of cyanide intoxication. The kit contains amyl nitrite inhalers, sodium nitrite ampules for injection, and sodium thiosulfate ampules for injection. The following instructions and chart may be used with the Lilly cyanide antidote kit. The manufacturer's package insert instructions may differ slightly from this procedure. All doses are given in milliliters.

N-acetylcysteine (Mucomyst) — traditionally employed as a mucolytic expectorant but has now demonstrated effectiveness in preventing hepatotoxicity resulting from acetaminophen overdose. It has recently been approved by the Food and Drug Administration for antidotal use. N-acetylcysteine is thought to be a surrogate for glutathione in the liver, since N-acetylcysteine is rich in sulfhydryl groups. Several protocols for oral and intravenous administration of the drug exist. The most successful to date is the 72-hour oral regimen of 140 mg/kg loading dose, followed by 17 doses at 4-hour intervals. The most effective intravenous course of therapy appears to be 140 mg/kg followed by 70 mg/kg maintenance every 4 hours for a total of 12 doses. If N-acetylcysteine is vomited by a patient, the dose must be repeated. If vomiting of a dose persists, it may be necessary to position a gastric tube in the duodenum and administer the N-acetylcysteine undiluted, as 10 or 20 percent solution. Antiemetic drugs may also be given, usually 30 minutes before a dose of N-acetylcysteine. Droperidol (Inapsine) has been used intravenously for this purpose at a dose of 1.25 mg, given 30 minutes before the dose of N-acetylcysteine.

Ethyl alcohol — one of the less toxic alcohols used as a competitive inhibitor of the metabolism of methyl alcohol and ethylene glycol, thus preventing the biotransformation of these compounds to formaldehyde and glyoxylic acid, respectively. Ethyl alcohol should be available as absolute alcohol for dilution to a 10 percent solution for intravenous use. A 50 percent solution may be used orally.

Methylene blue — chemically methylthionine chloride and an aniline derivative used to treat methemoglobinemia due to chemicals such as nitrates and nitrites. Its value is due to physiologic transformation to a reduced form known as leukomethylene blue (colorless), which is then again oxidized to methylene blue in the presence of methemoglobin. The methemoglobin is then converted to hemoglobin once again. Give at a dose of 1 to 2 mg/kg (0.1 to 0.2 ml/kg of a 1 percent solution). Do not use methylene blue to reverse methemoglobinemia in cyanide poisoning because it may induce the release of free cyanide ion.

TABLE 2-1: INSTRUCTIONS AND DOSES FOR USE WITH CYANIDE ANTIDOTE KIT

INITIAL INTRAVENOUS DOSE SODIUM NITRITE 3% WEIGHT (Kg)	INITIAL INTRAVENOUS DOSE SODIUM THIOSULFATE 25%	
	DOSE (ml) = 0.33 ml/kg	DOSE (ml) = 1.65 ml/kg
5	X 0.33 ml = 1.65	X 1.65 ml = 8.25
6	1.98	9.9
7	2.31	11.55
8	2.64	13.2
9	2.97	14.85
10	3.3	16.5
11	3.63	18.15
12	3.96	19.8
13	4.29	21.45
14	4.62	23.1
15	4.95	24.75
16	5.28	26.4
17	5.61	28.05
18	5.94	29.7
19	6.27	31.35
20	6.6	33.0
21	6.93	34.65
22	7.26	36.3
23	7.59	37.95
24	7.92	39.6
25	8.25	41.25

IN AN EMERGENCY WHEN 100 PERCENT OXYGEN IS BEING ADMINISTERED DO THE FOLLOWING:

1. Break one of the amyl nitrite inhalers into a handkerchief or gauze pad and hold in front of the patient's mouth for 30 seconds, rest for 30 seconds, reapply for 30 seconds, and repeat until the sodium nitrite ampule can be drawn up for injection. Stop once the sodium nitrite has been injected. Use a new inhaler every 3 minutes.
2. Inject the sodium nitrite intravenous push over 1 to 2 minutes according to the weight table above.
3. Immediately thereafter, through the same needle and vein, inject the sodium thiosulfate according to the weight table above.
4. If signs of poisoning reappear, repeat the above procedure at half the above doses.
5. See Lilly package insert for subsequent doses.

Naloxone (Narcan) — narcotic antagonist of choice used to reverse respiratory depression from narcotics and synthetic derivatives or analogs of narcotics. Do not use older narcotic antagonists, since only naloxone is inert in the absence of narcotics. The dose of naloxone required to treat overdosed patients may exceed manufacturer's recommended amount. An initial intravenous dose of 0.4 to 2 mg may be administered in adults. Initial dosing may be repeated at 3-minute intervals until respiratory function is stable. Children receive a starting dose of 0.01 mg/kg. If there is no response, give 0.1 mg/kg. In severe narcotic overdose, doses up to 4 mg have been used to reverse respiratory depression. Continuous intravenous infusion of naloxone has been used in adults at a rate 0.4 to 0.8 mg/hr.

Pralidoxime or 2-PAM (Protopam) — the only acetylcholinesterase reactivator currently available for general use in the United States. It is used in the management of acetylcholinesterase-inhibiting pesticides (e.g., the organophosphates). It is administered after atropine in life-threatening situations at a dose of 1 g intravenously, given over several minutes. Give children 250 mg per dose, slowly intravenously. Refer to package insert for repeat doses.

Physostigmine salicylate injection — itself a cholinesterase inhibitor, it is used to reverse the toxic effects of drugs producing anticholinergic crisis (e.g., atropine and other belladonna alkaloids), and for the cardiovascular and seizure effects of cyclic antidepressants, if more conventional drugs fail. A therapeutic trial of 0.5 mg may be given slowly intravenously. This drug must be titrated by dosing at 5-minute intervals up to a maximum of 2 mg. Repeat doses may be necessary after 1 hour.

Vitamin K — promotes the hepatic biosynthesis of prothrombin and other clotting factors and therefore is used to treat drug-induced hypoprothrombinemia. Anticoagulants such as warfarin and its congeners act as competitive antagonists of vitamin K and interfere with the biosynthesis of prothrombin and other clotting factors. The dose of vitamin K is high because it is a competitive antagonist for the poison, warfarin, in the liver. That is, the dose of vitamin K must be present in high enough concentrations to compete with the poison at its site of activity. Dose in warfarin poisoning is 1 to 5 mg intramuscularly in a child and 10 mg intramuscularly in an adult. Vitamin K_1 may be administered orally in the absence of vomiting.

Chelating Agents

Calcium disodium EDTA (edetate calcium disodium injection, USP, Calcium Disodium Versenate, $CaNa_2EDTA$).

Symptomatic children with acute encephalopathy — Administered intravenously, this chelate strongly enhances the mobilization and excretion of lead from the body. Lead displaces calcium ion from the molecular arrangement of the chelate. The dosage is 1,500 mg/m²/day. Four hours after the first dose of BAL (see below), start continuous infusion of CaNa₂EDTA, 1,500 mg/m²/day. Continue therapy with BAL and CaNa₂EDTA for 5 days. Interrupt therapy for 2 days. Treat for 5 additional days, including BAL if blood lead level remains high. Other cycles may be needed depending on blood lead rebound.

Symptomatic children without symptoms or signs of acute encephalopathy — 1,000 mg/m²/day. Four hours after the first dose of BAL (see below), start CaNa₂EDTA 1,000 mg/m²/day, preferably by continuous infusion, or in 6 divided doses intravenously (through a heparin lock). Continue therapy with CaNa₂EDTA for 5 days. Interrupt therapy for 2 days. Treat for 5 additional days, including BAL if blood lead level remains high. Other cycles may be needed depending on blood lead rebound.

BAL injection (British anti-lewisite, also called dimercaprol) — dimercaprol forms a stable chelate with a variety of metals, including lead, arsenicals, mercurials, gold salts, bismuth, chromium, nickel, and copper. It prevents inhibition of sulfhydryl enzymes by metals and also reactivates such enzymes.

Symptomatic children in danger of acute encephalopathy — 450 mg/m²/day. Start with 75 mg/m² intramuscularly every 4 hours.

Symptomatic children without symptoms or signs of acute encephalopathy — 300 mg/m²/day. Start with 50 mg/m² intramuscularly every 4 hours.

Penicillamine — an effective chelator of copper, zinc, mercury, and lead that promotes the excretion of these metals in the urine. The decided advantage over other chelating agents is that it can be given orally.

Deferoxamine — chelating agent with a remarkable affinity for ferric iron, used for acute iron poisoning. If the patient is not in shock, deferoxamine may be given intramuscularly at a dose of 90 mg/kg up to a maximum single dose of 1 g every 8 hours for 3 doses if serum iron exceeds total iron binding capacity (TIBC) or 500 micrograms/ml (see Chap. 13). Manufacturer's recommended dose is 1 g initially followed by 0.5 g every 4 hours for 2 doses. Depending on clinical response, administer subsequent doses of 0.5 g every 4 to 12 hours, not exceeding 6 g in 24 hours. Monitor urine for the characteristic red color if deferoxamine has been given, indicating chelated complex is being excreted. Deferoxamine may be stopped 24 hours after beginning therapy or sooner if urine loses reddish color, indicating a decrease in the concentration of the excreted chelate.

Supportive Drugs

Benztropine mesylate (Cogentin) — a longer-acting drug also used to treat extrapyramidal reactions caused by the phenothiazines. It has more side effects than diphenhydramine; although it may be used in adults, diphenhydramine is preferable in children (see below).

Diphenhydramine HCL (Benadryl) — used to treat acute extrapyramidal reactions to psychotropic drugs, particularly the phenothiazines. Administer 1 to 2 mg/kg/dose intravenously with a maximum single dose of 50 mg. Also used to pretreat patients who are hypersensitive to animal antivenins prepared from horse serum or who have developed serum sickness following their use. Use an intravenous dose of 50 mg every 2 to 4 hours, not to exceed 400 mg in 24 hours, in adults.

Lidocaine — for the treatment of ventricular arrhythmias. Loading dose (adult and child): administer 1 mg/kg/dose. Repeat a dose of 0.5 to 1 mg/kg 20 minutes later if needed. Maintenance dose (adult and child): Administer 10 to 40 micrograms/kg/min by continuous intravenous infusion. Begin maintenance dose concurrent with loading dose.

Phenytoin — for the treatment of ventricular arrhythmias. Loading dose (adult and child): Administer 15 mg/kg up to 1 g intravenously not to exceed a rate of 0.5 mg/kg/min. Maintenance dose (adult): 2 mg/kg intravenously every 12 hours as needed. Maintenance dose (child): 2 mg/kg intravenously every 8 hours as needed. Monitor serum phenytoin levels just before initiating and during maintenance therapy to ensure therapeutic levels of 10 to 20 microgram/ml.

Physostigmine — indications may include seizures, severe hallucinations, hypertension, and arrhythmias in the presence of anticholinergic symptoms *unresponsive* to standard anticonvulsant and antiarrhythmic agents. Coma may be reversed diagnostically, but do not give physostigmine continuously just to keep a patient awake. Adults: 1 to 2 mg slowly intravenously repeated in 20 minutes if symptoms are not reversed. Repeat the effective dose if life-threatening symptoms recur. Child: 0.5 mg slowly intravenously, repeated at 5-minute intervals until maximum dose of 2 mg has been given. Repeat maximum dose if life-threatening symptoms recur. Physostigmine is metabolized within 30 to 60 minutes, and repeated doses are often necessary.

Propranolol — Adult: 1 mg intravenously every 2 to 5 minutes until a response is seen or 10 mg has been given. Child: Dilute 1 mg of propranolol in 10 ml of saline or intravenous fluid to prepare a concentration of 0.1 mg/ml. Infuse 1 ml (0.1 mg of propranolol)/min of this dilution to the desired effect or until maximum calculated dose of 1 mg is reached. Repeat *only once* after 10 minutes if necessary.

Emetics

Syrup of ipecac — emetic of choice, reasonably "safe," oral, centrally acting drug used to induce vomiting. See the section on emergency treatment in this chapter for a detailed discussion.

Other emetics — Do not use sodium chloride (table salt), zinc sulfate, copper sulfate, and household remedies (e.g., mustard) to induce emesis. These substances are either ineffective, and consequently waste time, or are dangerous.

Adsorbents

Activated charcoal — destructive distillation of organic matter (e.g., coconut shells) tends to be molecularly disruptive so that increased surface area of the particles occurs in the manufacture of charcoal. However, additional, special treatment is required to "activate" the particle surface. Such activation is accomplished by treating the charcoal, at high temperature, with steam and carbon dioxide or other inert gases. Activated charcoal is administered in doses of 15 to 30 grams in children and 30 to 100 grams in adults. See the more detailed discussion on the administration of charcoal earlier in this chapter.

Cholestyramine — a resin that may have value as an adjunct in the treatment of lipid-soluble pesticide poisoning.

Castor oil — possibly effective as a ligand in complexing lipid-soluble drugs in the gastrointestinal tract. Used here as an adsorbent, not a laxative.

Cathartics

Sodium and **magnesium sulfate, magnesium citrate** (citrate of magnesia) — useful "saline" cathartics (laxatives). Because they are saline (soluble salts), they increase the amount of water in the bowel by osmosis, thus producing bulk. Catharsis usually occurs within 2 hours. Citrate of magnesia in children under 5 years: 4 ml/kg single dose. In children 5 to 12 years: 4 oz (120 ml) single dose. In adults: 10 oz (300 ml) single dose. Sodium and magnesium sulfate: 250 mg/kg/dose.

Antivenins and Biological Agents

Snake antivenin — Most antivenins are produced by hyperimmunization of horses. A high percentage of people who receive antivenin develop serum sickness. Antivenin is thus used only if there is evidence of systemic or severe local envenomation. Perform a preliminary intradermal or ophthalmic test of hypersensitivity (see Chap. 18). The dose of antivenin required may be very large, since neutralizing antibody titers of antivenins are much lower than those of most bacterial antitoxins. The crotalid or pit viper antivenin commercially available in the United States is produced against venoms of two species of North American rattlesnakes but is clinically effective against venoms of all North American pit vipers and probably most medically important tropical American species.

Black widow spider antivenin — Most healthy adults will survive a bite of a black widow spider (*Lactrodectus mactans*) with only supportive care. For patients over age 65 or under 12 or with underlying medical problems such as hypertension and cardiovascular disease, the antivenin is indicated. It is prepared from the serum of horses hyperimmunized with black widow spider venom. The dose is one vial of the reconstituted antivenin diluted in 50 ml of normal saline and infused over approximately 30 minutes. All the dangers associated with snake antivenin of similar origin apply to the use of black widow spider antivenin (see Chap. 18).

"Ion Trapping" Drugs

Certain water-soluble drugs that exhibit either acid or alkaline characteristics can be "trapped" in the urine following filtration by the renal glomeruli. This prevents reabsorption into the circulation, thus shortening the duration of effect of the drug.

References — Chapter 2

M. J. Bayer, and B. H. Rumack, *Poisoning and Overdose.* (Rockville, MD: Aspen Publications, 1983).

L. Chin, A. L. Picchioni, and W. M. Bourn, "Optimal Antidote Dose of Activated Charcoal." *Toxicol Appl Pharmacol.* 26:103-108, 1973.

R. H. Dreisback, *Handbook of Poisoning*, 11th ed., Los Altos, CA: Lange Med. Pub., 1983.

L. R. Goldfrank, *Toxicologic Emergencies*. (Norwalk, CT: Appleton-Century-Crofts Publishers, 1982).

K. Kulig, et al., "Management of Acutely Poisoned Patients Without Gastric Emptying." *Ann. Emerg. Med.* 14:562-567, 1985.

W. F. Lanphear, "Gastric Lavage." *J. Emerg. Med.* "4:43-47, 1986.

H. C. Mofenson, and J. Greensher, "The Unknown Poison." *Pediatr.* 54:336-342, 1974.

W. O. Robertson, "Syrup of ipecac. A Slow or Fast Emetic?" *Am. J. Dis. Child.* 103:136, 1962.

S. M. Pond, "Role of Repeated Oral Doses of Activated Charcoal in Clinical Toxicology." *Medical Toxicology.* 1:3-11, 1986.

B. H. Rumack, ed., "Poisindex Information System, Micromedex: General or Unknown Poison Management." *Management* 47:14-C1, 1986.

B. H. Rumack, cd., "Poisindex Information System, Micromedex: General Toxicology Information Management." *Management* 50:14-I1, 1986.

CHAPTER 3 *BASIC TOXICOLOGY*

The absorption, distribution, biotransformation, and excretion of drugs and toxins, coupled with dosage and interactions, determine the concentration of a drug or a toxin at the site of action and thus the intensity of the effects as a function of time.

Pharmacokinetics relates specifically to the variations with time of drug and toxin concentrations, particularly in the blood, serum, and plasma. By extrapolation, the concentration of a drug or toxin may be interpreted in terms of drug or toxin effect, i.e., by pharmacodynamics.

The fundamental principle of pharmacokinetics is based on the most elementary kinetic model. The distribution of a drug or toxin is assumed to be relatively uniform and to occur rapidly relative to absorption and elimination. For this model the volume of distribution of a drug is that in which it would appear to be distributed during the steady state if it existed throughout that volume at the same concentration as in plasma:

$$Vd = \frac{\text{Total amount of drug in body}}{\text{Concentration of drug in plasma}}$$

Vd is the volume distribution, and absorption and elimination of the drug are assumed to follow exponential first-order kinetics; that is, a constant portion of drug present is eliminated per unit of time. As one can imagine, the concentration in blood or plasma will vary with administration of a single dose or repeated doses, which will result in accumulation.

ABSORPTION

The absorption of drugs and toxins through different portals of entry (e.g., gastrointestinal tract, subcutaneous tissue, muscle, and skin) must be discussed.

Absorption of substances after ingestion depends on the substance ingested and on the secretory state and emptying time of the stomach. Small, neutral, water-soluble molecules such as alcohol (and water itself) are absorbed rapidly from the stomach, with the amount limited mostly by the stomach's emptying time. Absorption of other agents varies with their lipid solubility, depending on the stomach's secretory state. For example, aspirin, a weak acid, is almost entirely unionized in lipid-soluble form at the pH of the secreting stomach and is therefore well absorbed. However, when aspirin is given with an alkali, the fraction present as a water- soluble salt increases and absorption is then as slow as in the small intestine. On the other hand, water solubility increases and thus determines the rate of absorption for subcutaneously and intramuscularly administered substances.

The skin, like mucosae, conforms to the lipid barrier model with pores for water-soluble substances. In other words, the more lipid soluble a substance is, the better it is absorbed. The keratin layer of the skin diminishes absorption through skin as compared with absorption through mucosae.

DISTRIBUTION

The free distribution of agents within the body is hindered by numerous membranes. Although blood flow, albumin binding, and differential distribution are important, the basic unit is the cell or plasma membrane. The cell membrane is a lipoprotein that also complies, like skin and mucosae, to the lipid barrier with pores model. Thus cell membranes are permeable to lipid- soluble molecules and impermeable to polar water-soluble molecules. In addition, they contain pores for the passage of water-soluble substances such as water itself, urea, and alcohol. These membranes also have channels for carrier-facilitated transport, as discussed later. The transfer across cell membranes can therefore be passive by filtration, by diffusion, or by carrier protein facilitation. Transport across these membranes can also be active when energy is required, which is generated by adenosinetriphosphatase (ATPase).

Blood flow also influences the transport of a substance to specific areas of the body; highly vascular areas have a higher drug or toxic agent level than poorly vascularized areas. Some substances such as sulfonamides are significantly plasma albumin bound. The albumin complex dissociates freely and is of some but usually little practical significance except on binding a substance. Bilirubin may be dissociated from albumin, thus increasing the level of bilirubin and causing significant hyperbilirubinemia in newborns and other persons with borderline elevation of bilirubin.

The differential distribution of substances into a particular compartment (e.g., the brain, liver, or adipose tissue) follows specialized patterns. The blood-brain barrier refers to the fact that the capillaries in the brain are lipid permeable, with pores for water-soluble agents, but cannot filter plasma freely into interstitial spaces because the interstitial spaces are small and the supporting lipid-permeable glial cells are in close opposition to the capillary wall. Hence quaternary ammonium derivatives such as curare and acetylcholine, which exist entirely in salt form at body pH and are water soluble but lipid insoluble, do not penetrate the blood-brain barrier.

Substances with high intrinsic lipid solubility and low water solubility may accumulate in high concentration in adipose tissues (e.g., thiopental and the chlorinated hydrocarbon insecticides). Substances also accumulate at the sites of metabolism and excretion — the liver if it is the site of biotransformation, the intestine if secretion is into the bile, and the kidney if the metabolites are concentrated in tubular urine.

The distribution of drugs and toxins across the placenta is a difficult and incompletely studied problem. The fetal tissues covering the villi are in contact with maternal blood. Some substances move back and forth across this membrane as if conforming to the lipid barrier model. As expected, the general anesthetic agents, the narcotic analgesics, and the barbiturates reach and depress the fetal nervous system, whereas quaternary ammonium compounds such as succinylcholine do not.

Whether drugs or toxins will appear in breast milk can be predicted by the lipid barrier model. Lipid solubility favors transport; since milk is slightly more acidic than plasma, basic compounds such as erythromycin are concentrated in milk. Small neutral molecules such as alcohol appear in milk in the same concentration as in plasma, and acidic drugs such as penicillin appear in milk in concentrations less than in plasma.

TERMINATION OF ACTION

The action of substances may be terminated by several mechanisms, including biotransformation, excretion, redistribution, repair of drug-induced changes, physiologic compensation, and interaction of agents.

Biotransformation

Biotransformation modifies the effects of chemical agents in several ways, such as forming an inactive metabolite from an active one, the most common mechanism; forming an active metabolite from an initially inactive compound; forming an active metabolite from an initially active compound; and forming a toxic metabolite from an initially less toxic compound.

The major organ where these reactions occur is the liver, both in the mitochondrial and the microsomal fractions. The important reactions that substances undergo during biotransformation are conjugation, oxidation, hydrolysis, and hydrogenation or reduction. All these reactions, except conjugation, are chemically self-explanatory.

Conjugation includes a variety of chemical reactions such as alkylation, esterification, and so forth in which there is a combination of a drug or toxin with a highly polar ionic moiety, thus increasing the water solubility of the original compound, which can then be rapidly eliminated. Some conjugation reactions are glucuronidation, acetylation, sulfation, and methylation as well as glycine and glutamine conjugation.

In *glucuronidation* the activated glucuronic acid reacts with a phenolic or an alcoholic hydroxyl group to form an ether glucuronide or, with a carboxylic acid, to form an ester glucuronide (e.g., diethylstilbestrol).

In *sulfation* phenols, alcohols, and aromatic amines can be converted to sulfates or sulfanilic acid derivatives by an active sulfate provided by adenosine-3-phosphate-5-phosphosulfate (e.g., sulfonamides).

In *methylation* a methyl group from S-adenosylmethionine converts a phenolic or alcoholic hydroxyl group to a methoxy group (O-methylation, e.g., epinephrine), or a hydrogen of an amine converts the parent compound into a quaternary amine (N-methylation, e.g., histamine).

In *acetylation* the acetyl group of acetyl coenzyme A replaces a hydrogen of an amine or amide group (e.g., isoniazid). Glycine and glutamine may also conjugate with acids (e.g., the conversion of aspirin to salicyluric acid is by glycine conjugation).

Oxidation reactions occur mostly in the liver microsomes (smooth endoplasmic reticulum) and also in the hepatic mitochondria. Hepatic microsomal oxidases convert lipid-soluble substances to more easily excreted and less active water-soluble metabolites. Before conjugation, the first step in the process is usually hydroxylation. Hydroxylation of aromatic rings or alkyl side chains occurs at cytochrome P-450. Then oxygen is activated by nicotinamide adenine dinucleotide, and the drug is oxidized. There is little substrate specificity beyond the requirement that the foreign substance be lipid soluble. The activity of these enzymes is increased or induced during the administration of many long-acting, lipid-soluble compounds such as phenobarbital, phenytoin, and chlorinated hydrocarbon insecticides.

Other oxidative enzymes also important in the metabolism of a relatively few specific compounds are alcohol dehydrogenase of the liver mitochondria, which converts ethanol and a few other alcohols to their corresponding aldehyde; aldehyde dehydrogenase, which converts the resulting aldehyde to the corresponding acid (see Chap. 8); xanthine oxidase, which governs the final steps in the synthesis of uric acid; monoamine oxidase of mitochondria, which converts simple monoamines to their aldehydes; and diamine oxidase of mitochondria, which diaminates compounds with two amines.

Hydrolytic enzymes such as proteases, peptidases, phosphatases, acetylcholinesterases, and esterases are important. Esters such as procaine and meperidine are examples of drugs that are esters whose activity is destroyed by hydrolysis. The inactivation of penicillin G depends on the hydrolytic opening of the lactam ring.

Excretion

Gases and volatile industrial solvents and drugs such as alcohol and paraldehyde are absorbed and excreted across the pulmonary alveolar membrane. Although they may have other more important routes of excretion or metabolism, their content in alveolar air reflects plasma levels in a consistent way and can be used to quantify the degree of intoxication.

Drug toxins and their metabolites or conjugates appear in the urine in the glomerular filtrate, and a greater or lesser fraction is then reabsorbed through the tubular cell. The more lipid soluble the material, the greater the degree of reabsorption; the more water soluble the material, the greater the fraction remaining in the urine. Thus, the excretion of drugs and toxins can be altered by either acidification or alkalinization of the urine. For example, intoxication with weak acids such as salicylates and barbiturates is treated by maintaining a high volume of alkaline urine because weak acids exist largely in the salt-ionized, water-soluble form, and reabsorption is greatly decreased.

The renal tubule is also able to transport actively or secrete organic anions and cations through separate channels. For example, excretion of penicillin is by tubular secretion. Furthermore, drugs and their conjugates may appear in the intestinal content after being secreted in the bile or excreted by the colon. Specific substances may also appear in saliva and sweat in significant amounts.

Redistribution

The differential distribution of a substance, which depends to a great extent on its solubility and the blood flow to different tissues, may be a mechanism for terminating its activity. For example, intravenous thiopental produces a high plasma level immediately carried to the brain by the cerebral blood flow. Subsequently, the poorly perfused adipose tissue slowly takes up enough thiopental to bring about its withdrawal from the brain and its termination of action.

Repair of Drug-induced Changes

Some agents disappear from the body after a few hours but cause changes that may take many days for correction. For example, after prothrombin synthesis is inhibited by a coumarin anticoagulant such as warfarin rat poison, the effect persists until new protein is synthesized by the liver.

Physiologic Compensation

Compensation by the organism may either decrease or completely abolish the effects of a drug or may modify certain responses such as pulse rate or blood pressure and give the impression of a decreased overall response. For example, the compensatory reflexes originating from a change in blood pressure whenever a pressor or depressor drug is given cannot modify a drug-induced rise in pressure but may cause a reflex bradycardia that can obscure the drug's primary effect. Another example is vasoconstrictor drugs such as norepinephrine and ephedrine, which can reduce cardiac output enough to limit the rise in blood pressure caused by their vasoconstrictive action. The reduced response of the blood pressure when vasoconstricting and other actions are maximal is called *tachyphylaxis*.

Tolerance of a qualitatively different kind follows the administration of organic nitrates and the narcotic analgesics. In this case, not only must larger and larger doses be given to maintain the effect, but also normally lethal doses can be given without danger or even much effect.

Interaction of Agents

Drugs and toxins administered simultaneously or sequentially may act independently of each other or may interact to diminish or augment the expected response, causing unanticipated toxicity.

The major types of drug interaction are addition, antagonism, interference with absorption, displacement of protein-binding sites, chemical combination, stimulation or inhibition of drug metabolism, interaction at receptor site, and stimulation or inhibition of excretion.

The most common type of drug interaction is simple addition of effects, such as when a patient taking barbiturates also takes alcohol. The effect of a chemical may also be terminated by giving its competitive or physiologic antagonist. For example, the effect of morphine can be antagonized by nalorphine, the effect of histamine by epinephrine, and the effect of anticholinergic drugs by physostigmine.

When certain drugs and foods are given orally without an adequate interval between their administration, they may interfere with the absorption of each other and therefore with the effective dose. For example, tetracyclines chelate divalent cations such as magnesium and the calcium present in milk or an antacid and therefore are themselves less absorbed. Phenytoin, phenobarbital, and oral contraceptives interfere with folate deconjugase and thereby prevent the release of folic acid from polyglutamates and result in folic acid deficiency.

Drugs may also be reversibly bound to plasma protein during transport and may compete for binding sites, displacing either each other or bilirubin. For example, warfarin is displaced by acids such as sulfonamides and phenylbutazone.

Agents may combine chemically in plasma and in the extracellular fluid. For example, heparin is neutralized by protamine and fluoride by calcium.

As previously mentioned, hepatic microsomal oxidases govern the metabolism of numerous drugs. Many lipid-soluble drugs and toxins can stimulate the enzymatic activity of these hepatic microsomial oxidases. For example, the same dosage of a coumarin anticoagulant and of phenobarbital give lower plasma levels and have a lesser physiologic effect if the patient is also taking glutethimide, meprobamate, phenytoin, griseofulvin, 3 4-benzpyrene, or corticosteroids.

Some drugs such as monoamine oxidase inhibitors and xanthine oxidase inhibitors act by inhibiting the enzyme responsible for the metabolism of some endogenous substance. When a drug or toxin related to that endogenous substance is administered, the exogenous compound may not be destroyed and may cause an intense reaction. For example, after monoamine oxidase inhibitors are given, the effects of agents such as tyramine, present in cheese, red wine, and other fermented foods, is intensified. A more common example of inhibition of drug metabolism is the toxicity of alcohol by alcohol dehydrogenase inhibitors such as disulfiram and nitrofurantoin.

Interaction at receptor sites by agonists and antagonists is sometimes less easily anticipated. For example, the antihypertensive guanethidine is antagonized by other compounds that block norepinephrine uptake such as antipsychotic and antidepressant drugs.

A substance may also either inhibit or facilitate excretion of another substance. For example, many acidic drugs and their metabolites share the same pathway of secretion and reabsorption in the renal tubule. Thus, probenecid may prolong the action of penicillin by blocking its tubular secretion.

TOXICOLOGY OF DRUGS

Adverse reactions to drugs are caused by overdose, side effects, allergy, idiosyncrasy, and developmental problems.

Overdose is the expected undesirable effect of a drug because of the large dose administered (e.g., cardiac arrhythmia caused by a large dose of digitalis).

Side effects are undesirable effects of a drug that can and do happen with predictable frequency even when a usual dose of a drug is given (e.g., diarrhea is a common side effect after administration of ampicillin).

Allergic reaction is an undesirable effect (or effects) caused by antibodies produced by the host against a particular drug (e.g., anaphylaxis caused by penicillin).

Idiosyncrasy is an undesirable effect of a drug, thought to be unpredictable, for which there is no acceptable, conclusive explanation, other than a possible genetic defect. For example, certain people taking sulfonamide drugs develop a sensitivity rash when they are exposed to light; and hemolysis occurs in individuals who are deficient in glucose-6-phosphate dehydrogenase (G-6-PD) when they are exposed to oxidizing drugs and chemicals such as primaquine and naphthalene.

Developmental adverse reactions are reactions certain

drugs cause that are directly related to the patient's level of developmental maturation (e.g., tetracycline, if given to a pregnant woman, will stain the fetus' developing teeth).

Nonallergic Reactions

In the understanding and control of all adverse reactions, except possibly allergic and idiosyncratic reactions, the first step is to conduct animal studies. Animal toxicity studies must precede trials of new drugs in human beings. The relative sensitivity of different animals poses a problem. For example, rats and cats may be 10 times, and dogs as much as 6 times, more sensitive than humans to certain chemicals and drugs. Nevertheless, the data do have predictive value and must be collected. Animal toxicity studies can be described as acute, subacute, and chronic.

Acute toxicity is measured by the median lethal dose (LD_{50}) observed during the first 14 days. This is the dose that will kill 50 percent of a group of animals under stated conditions. The LD_{50} is an assay, not an absolute measurement. The experimental conditions must be standardized. Both the species and the strain of the animals should be recorded, as well as the route of administration, the vehicle in which the drug is dissolved or suspended, and the concentration and volume of the solution injected. Because diet, ambient temperature, season, and other variables are difficult to control, a standard related drug should be studied for comparison and 4 species must be used, including 1 nonrodent. The routes of administration must be those that will be used in humans.

Subacute toxicity experiments are usually the second step in preclinical toxicity testing. These tests extend for 14 to 21 days and establish the minimal toxic and maximal tolerated dose as well as the possible role of accumulation and tolerance.

In **chronic toxicity** experiments the drug is given to animals of 2 species for 90 days in at least 3 dosage levels, one of which is the predicted therapeutic level and one the level at which at least minimal toxicity occurs. Growing animals are used for this test. Weight gain during the experiment is compared with that of a control group. Postmortem examinations are done at the conclusion of the experiment. The chronic toxicity test in dogs should continue for 1 year.

Afterward, the drug is ready for human trial, which is divided into three phases. In phase I the drug is given to healthy adult volunteers to determine dose, duration of action, and toxicity. In phase II the drug is tested for its specific therapeutic effects in limited clinical trials, and in phase III the drug is used in clinical trials designed to establish the value of the drug under conditions of actual practice.

Frequently, absolute toxicity is less important than the ratio between the toxic and the therapeutic doses. The median effective dose (ED_{50}) is the dose that is therapeutically effective in 50 percent of a population similar to that on which the median lethal dose (LD_{50}) was determined. The ratio $LD_{50}:ED_{50}$ is the therapeutic index. Because the physician hopes to avoid even one fatality due to direct drug toxicity, the dosage that produces the first dangerous toxic sign is often of greater importance than the therapeutic index.

Allergic Reactions

As previously mentioned, most adverse reactions to drugs and toxins are related to the amount taken or administered. The properties of the particular substance determine the exact nature of the toxic effect. A given patient may be more or less sensitive to a particular effect, but all individuals respond if a dose is great enough.

In contrast, allergic or hypersensitivity reactions depend on the patient's reactivity altered by prior contact with the drug or toxin that functions as an allergen or antigen. The manifestations of allergic reactions are unrelated to the pharmacologic effect of the drug or toxin and resemble those of other allergic reactions.

Most drugs and toxins, except some animal toxins that are protein, cannot function as complete antigens but only as haptens or partial antigens that must react with some homologous protein after administration. The altered body protein is antigenic, and the haptenic drug confers specificity. Penicillin is a well-studied example of a drug with a metabolite, penicillanic acid, that may function as a hapten.

Since not all reactions to drugs and toxins are immunochemical, one or more of the following criteria should be met to establish the allergic nature of an adverse reaction: circulating or cellular antibodies to the suspect drug, known immediate or delayed allergic pattern, reproduction of the reaction after recovery by a single test dose, occurrence of the reaction after a sensitizing period, lack of relationship to dosage level, and symptomatic relief by sympathomimetic amines, antihistamines, or anti-inflammatory steroids.

Idiosyncratic reactions are undesirable and previously unpredictable effects of a drug. In some cases these reactions can now be predicted because they are understood to be due to an enzymatic defect, such as G-6-PD deficiency, as mentioned above. G-6-PD deficiency is a genetic disorder seen in about 10 percent of American black males and fewer black females. It is also seen in low frequency among people of Mediterranean descent, such as Italians, Greeks, Arabs, and Sephardic Jews. The deficiency is responsible for destabilizing glutathione, a universal component of living cells. Lowered levels of glutathione make red blood cells particularly susceptible to hemolysis by oxidizing drugs and chemicals. In clinical studies involving instances of this type of reaction, instability of glutathione has been demonstrated in the erythrocytes of susceptible persons. This susceptibility is a *heightened* reaction or sensitivity, since a large enough dose of the substance would harm *all* people.

Other idiosyncratic reactions, such as some of the drug-induced blood dyscrasias, are still poorly understood and may even be allergic in nature.

Allergic reactions to drugs and toxins can be divided, like all allergic reactions, into immediate and delayed reactions.

Immediate. Immediate allergic reactions depend on the formation of immunoglobulins of the IgE class. The IgE or reaginic- or tissue-fixed antibody specific for the hapten is bound to the surface of tissue mast cells. When the substance is subsequently reintroduced, the sensitized cells are degranulated by the reaction of antigen and antibody on their surface, releasing histamine and other substances and most typically causing anaphylaxis or urticaria. Antibodies of the IgG and IgM classes are also formed and play a role in some immediate allergic reactions such as serum sickness and vasculitis. The word *immediate* is applicable because classically the reaction to the skin test appears within minutes in those individuals in whom it is positive.

Anaphylaxis is the most dangerous drug reaction. Delay in recognition and treatment increases the possibility of death. Anaphylaxis, unlike most other allergic reactions, can be produced and studied in animals. In anaphylaxis, histamine and other substances are released by mast cell degranulation, resulting in bronchiolar constriction presenting an asthmalike picture, i.e., localized edema of the larynx and glottal regions that may cause respiratory obstruction and vasodilation leading to hypotension and shock.

Urticaria and **angioneurotic edema** are caused more often by food allergens than by drugs and toxins. Urticaria (hives) is an acute inflammation of the skin characterized by erythematous, sharply demarcated, red elevated patches that are very pruritic. Angioneurotic edema is a giant urticaris involving the face and larynx. Some drugs such as morphine and its relatives are also able to liberate histamine by direct action on mast cells, producing nonallergic urticaria.

Serum sickness occurs after exposure to the offending drug following an incubation period of 5 to 14 days. Then a sudden decrease in the amount of circulating antibodies and deposition of antigen-antibody complex in the blood vessels occurs, resulting in fever, skin rash, adenopathy, and arthralgia that persist for several days.

Drug fever is another variant of serum sickness in which there is high fever for 1 to 3 weeks after the use of a drug. The fever usually persists for 2 to 3 days after the drug is discontinued.

Asthma and **rhinitis** due to drugs and toxins are rare and usually occur in patients with other allergies. Aspirin, sulfonamides, and penicillin have all been implicated in producing asthma and allergic rhinitis.

Systemic vasculitis resembling polyarteritis nodosa has been induced by drugs such as penicillin.

Autoimmune reactions may or may not be considered immediate allergic reactions; in many instances the exact mechanism is poorly understood. Thrombocytopenia due to quinidine administration, disseminated lupus erythematosus due to hydralazine administration, and drug-induced Coombs' positive hemolytic anemia are examples of such reactions.

Delayed. In the development of delayed hypersensitivity reactions, the drug (hapten)-protein combination is identified by the lymphocytes as foreign. The inflammatory process is precipitated by a delayed reaction, as in the tuberculin skin test, and reaches a peak only after 24 to 48 hours.

Drug-induced cutaneous reactions due to drugs acting as antigens after systemic administration can cause many skin reactions. Clinically, the reaction may be a minor morbilliform rash, resemble eczematous dermatitis, or progress to exfoliative dermatitis (erythema multiforme).

Some agranulocytoses caused by drugs are characterized by aplastic bone marrow and no antileukocyte antibodies, and the mechanism is not well understood (see aplastic anemia). Other cases of agranulocytosis are due to the abrupt peripheral destruction of granulocytes and are associated with cellular marrow and antileukocyte antibodies. These cases are considered allergic.

In aplastic anemia no causative mechanism has been established, but an association with certain agents is clear. The most common offenders are chloramphenicol, phenylbutazone, gold salts, and certain chlorinated hydrocarbons. The condition is one of bone marrow depression. Recovery is very slow, and mortality is high. However, the condition may be reversed if detected early.

References — Chapter 3

R. Baer, and V. H. Witten, "Drug Eruptions." *Year Book of Dermatology*. 9:37, 1960-61.

T. B. Binns, ed., *Absorption and Distribution of Drugs.* (London: Longman, 1964).

M. R. Boyd, "Biochemical Mechanisms in Chemical-Induced Injury." *Critical Rev. Toxicol.* 7:103, 1980.

A. H. Conney, "Pharmacological Implications of Microsomal Enzyme Induction." *Pharmacol. Rev.* 19:317, 1967.

P. D. Hansten, *Drug Interactions*. (Philadelphia: Lea & Febiger, 1971).

C. M. Huguley, Jr., "Hematological Reactions." *J.A.M.A.* 196:408, 1966.

L. P. James, Jr., and K. F. Austen, "Fatal Systemic Anaphylaxis in Man." *N. Engl. J. Med.* 270:597, 1964.

B. N. LaDu, H. G. Mandel, and E. L. Way, *Fundamentals of Drug Metabolism and Disposition.* (Baltimore: Williams & Wilkins, 1971).

L. M. Lichtenstein, and P. S. Norman, "Human Allergic Reactions." *Am. J. Med.* 46:163, 1969.

H. Remmer, "The Role of the Liver in Drug Metabolism." *Am. J. Med.* 49:617, 1970.

J. W. Smith, L. G. Seidle, and L. E. Cluff, "Studies on the Epidemiology of Adverse Drug Reactions. Clinical Factors Influencing Susceptibility." *Ann. Intern. Med.* 65:629, 1966.

R. O. Wallerstein, et al., "Statewide Study of Chloramphenicol Therapy and Fatal Aplastic Anemia." *J.A.M.A.* 208:2045, 1969.

H. E. Whipple, ed., "Evaluation and Mechanisms of Drug Toxicity." *Ann. N. Y. Acad. Sci.* 123:1, 1965.

CHAPTER 4 *DIAGNOSTIC TOXICOLOGY*

Poisoning must be considered in any disease state of questionable etiology. As in any other clinical situation, the most important tools are the history and physical examination. Approach the differential diagnosis in an organized and rational fashion. The laboratory, either as a screening bedside tool or as a definitive quantitative measurement, can assist greatly.

DIFFERENTIAL DIAGNOSIS

When confronted with a poisoned patient, consider six general categories: gases, metals, inorganic nonmetals, volatiles, solvents, and nonvolatile organic substances.

Gases. Some toxic gases are hydrogen cyanide, carbon monoxide, and hydrogen sulfide. The very toxic hydrogen cyanide produces immediate tachypnea, shock, convulsion, and coma with red skin resembling that produced by carboxyhemoglobin. Carbon monoxide produces headache, confusion, and the typical cherry-red skin color due to carboxyhemoglobin. Hydrogen sulfide can be detected readily by the rotten egg odor emanating from the lungs and the greenish discoloration of the viscera.

Metals. Some toxic metals are lead, arsenic, mercury, cadmium, and zinc. Most metals cause multiorgan involvement, with definite involvement of the kidney and also of the gastrointestinal tract, brain, and other organ systems (see Chap. 20).

Inorganic nonmetals. Inorganic nonmetals are divided into acids (sulfuric acid), bases (ammonia and sodium hydroxide), oxidants (chlorates), and reducers (sulfides). They have different systemic effects but are mainly corrosive, with the principal effect in the upper gastrointestinal tract, i.e., esophageal burns (see Chap. 16).

Volatiles. Volatile substances, such as those which can be extracted by acid distillation (e.g., alcohol, ether, and cyanide) and those which can be extracted by alkaline distillation (e.g., aniline and amphetamine), have specific clinical manifestations (see Chaps. 6 and 7).

Solvents. Solvents are alcohol, acetone, benzene, and so forth. When a solvent is the suspected poison, some can be identified in blood and urine, such as alcohol and acetone, and some only in urine, such as benzene. However, the best method to diagnose solvent poisoning is breath analysis, which can be diagnostic hours to weeks after exposure (see Chaps. 8 and 15).

Nonvolatile organic substances. Substances that can be extracted by organic solvent, by acid extraction (barbiturates and aspirin), and by alkaline extraction (plant alkaloids) also have specific signs and symptoms (see Chaps. 6, 8, 11, and 17).

LABORATORY IN TOXICOLOGY

The clinical laboratory is always an important tool in the management of the poisoned patient. This section discusses some common tests and their basic principles. Toxicologic tests can be simple chemical colorimetric and fluorometric tests, spectrophotometric tests such as atomic absorption and ultraviolet, chromatographic tests such as paper, thin-layer, and gas, and immunochemical tests.

Simple chemical tests. Several simple colorimetric and fluorometric tests are useful to clinical toxicologists. The presence of barbiturates can be determined either by the mercury bichloride, diphenyl thiocarbazone (dithione) test or by the cobalt acetate isopropyl amine test.

A screening test for the presence of salicylates is the addition of a few drops of ferric chloride to the urine or gastric content. A more specific test that the clinical laboratory can perform for salicylate is the quantitative mercury bichloride ferric nitrate test.

The presence of phenothiazine in serum, urine, and gastric content can be determined by the screening ferric chloride test and by the more specific ferric chloride perchloric acid nitric acid test.

The presence of tricyclic antidepressants in serum, urine, and gastric content can be determined by the sulfuric acid-perchloric acid-nitric acid test.

The presence of several metals such as mercury, arsenic, antimony, and bismuth can be determined by Reinsch's test, namely, by depositing the metal on a copper wire when boiled.

Fluorometric tests are useful to determine the presence or absence of a block in the synthesis of hemoglobin, e.g., as it occurs in lead poisoning. Fluoresence can be elicited and measured when blood coproporphyrin is elevated by the addition to the blood of acetic acid, ether, and iodine, or acetic acid, ether, and hydrogen peroxide. Another fluorometric test that has replaced the coproporphyrin test is the test measuring the amount of free erythrocyte protoporphyrin (FEP). Of course other disease processes, such as iron deficiency anemia, will elevate FEP.

The presence of carbon monoxide can be detected by diluting blood with water to obtain a pink solution and then adding sodium hydroxide. If carbon monoxide is present, the solution will not change immediately to a straw color because carboxyhemoglobin is more resistant than hemoglobin to alkaline denaturation.

The presence of alcohol can be easily determined by breath analysis as previously described, by a simple chemical colorimetric test, by microdiffusion, and by steam distillation.

The presence of methemoglobin can be detected by adding potassium cyanide to the chocolate-colored blood (methemoglobin), which will turn the blood pink again.

In iron intoxication there are two simple chemical parts: the potassium ferrocyanide (Prussian blue) test and the thioglycolic acid-tripyridyl triazine colorimetric test.

Spectrometric tests. Several spectrometric tests, such as atomic absorption spectrometry and ultraviolet spectrophotometry, are useful tools in clinical toxicology.

Atomic absorption. The atomic absorption test after acid digestion is a very useful test for many metals, including lead, copper, cadmium, thallium, antimony, zinc, bismuth, barium, mercury, and iron. The atomic absorption test is based on the absorption of part of the light spectrum by different atoms during spectrophotometry.

Ultraviolet spectrophotometry. Ultraviolet spectrophotometry is based on the principle that many drugs, chemicals, and poisons show characteristic absorption curves with maximum or minimum peaks in the ultraviolet region of the spectrum. Ultraviolet spectrophotometry is rapid and gives a permanent record, but numerous drugs do not have a strong ultraviolet spectrum and the sensitivity is limited because several drugs have similar ultraviolet spectrums.

Chromatographic tests. Chromatography is a useful technique based on the differential migration of substances carried by a solvent through an absorbent layer of either paper (paper chromatography) or glass coated with flexible silica (silica gel chromatography).

Before chromatography is performed, the substance must be extracted from the particular body fluid or tissue with either an organic solvent or an ion exchange column. Then the extracted substance is allowed to migrate through the absorbent carried by the solvent or developer. One of the most commonly used developers is ethyl acetate methanol ammonia. To test for specific substances in specific techniques other solvents are used, such as toluene for marijuana.

Each specific substance is identified after the spot is stained by the distance it migrates (Rf), which is calculated by the following formula:

$$Rf = \frac{\text{distance traveled by drug}}{\text{distance traveled by solvent}}$$

Specific drugs and substances are stained by primary amines (amphetamines), iodoplatinate for tertiary amines (morphine, mercury sulfate), dithiocarbamate for barbiturates and glutethimide, methoxybenzene diammonium chloride for marijuana, and sulfuric acid for phenothiazines and antihistamines.

Thin-layer and paper chromatography. Thin-layer and paper chromatography are cheap and reliable tests, but they are not specific; that is, two drugs with similar Rf or which are picked up by the same chemical group cannot be separated. Furthermore, drugs take at least 4 hours to migrate.

Gas chromatography. Gas chromatography is another chromatographic technique that is used increasingly. In gas chromatography, extraction substances are boiled to a gas state and then carried through a column (fixed phase) of either solid or liquid by a carrier gas. Each specific substance has a different retention time. The technique is accurate and rapid, and it is simple to determine volatile compounds. However, like thin-layer and paper chromatography, its sensitivity varies somewhat, since separation of substances lies within the rate at which molecules in a gas state can be moved. Electron capturing measures each molecule. A further sophistication of the technique, making it the best available technique at present, is to follow gas chromatography with mass spectrometry. In mass spectrometry, after substances are placed through gas chromatography, each molecule is bombarded with high-energy electrons and the produced ions are then accelerated through a magnetic field. Each ion moves according to its mass.

Immunologic assay. Immunologic assay is yet another technique to identify drugs. All immunoassays are based on the production of antibody followed by competitive displacement of labeled drugs from the antibody complex by an unlabeled drug, as illustrated by the following equation:

$$Ab\ D^* + Ab\ D + D^*$$
$$Ab = antibody$$
$$D^* = labeled\ drug$$
$$D = unlabeled\ drug$$

Fundamental to the immunoassay technique is the coupling of a drug (hapten) with a carrier protein to form an antigenic complex used to stimulate in an animal-specific antibody production. Subsequently, the antibody is allowed to react with mixtures of labeled and unlabeled drugs. This reaction is called *competitive binding*. In it, the labeled drug is liberated from the antibody-labeled drug complex, and the quantity of liberated drug can be measured. The labeling system varies. It can be an active enzyme (lysozyme) in the enzyme multiplied immunoassay (EMIT); tanned red blood cells in hemagglutination (HI); a nitroxide molecule in the free radical assay technique (FRAT), and a labeled isotope in radioimmunoassay (RIA).

Immunoassays are useful because they require no extraction, but reliability depends greatly on the quality of the antibodies produced; in other words, the specificity depends on the specificity of the antibody. The detector system also influences the result.

For example, FRAT and EMIT are faster but not as sensitive as RIA and HI. Both RIA and FRAT require more expensive equipment than EMIT and HI.

References — Chapter 4

G. L. Berg, ed., *Farm Chemicals Handbook*. Annual publication (Willoughby, OH: Meister, 1986).

J. Doull, et al., *Toxicology*, 2nd ed. (New York: MacMillan, 1980).

S. Kaye, "Bedside Toxicology (Methods of Analysis)." *Pediatr. Clin. North Am.* 17:515-524, 1970.

T. A. Loomis, *Essentials of Toxicology*, 3rd ed. (Philadelphia: Lea & Febiger, 1978).

G. Morrison, and W. F. Durham, "Analytical Diagnosis of Pesticide Poisoning." *J.A.M.A.* 216:298-300, 1971.

F. G. Mullick, R. M. Drake, and N. S. Irey, "Adverse Reactions to Drugs: A Clinicopathologic Survey of 200 Infants and Children." *J. Pediatr.* 82:506-510, 1973.

I. Sunshine, *Handbook of Analytical Toxicology.* (Cleveland, OH: Chemical Rubber Publishing Co., 1971).

J. A. Thomas, M. G. Mawhinney, and G. R. Knotts, "Substances with Potential for Abuse by Elementary and Secondary School Pupils." *Clin. Pediatr.* 12:17A-36A, 1973.

U. S. National Institute of Occupational Safety and Health, *Toxic Substances List.* (Washington, DC: U. S. Government Printing Office, 1972).

DRUG POISONING AND OVERDOSE

Pharmaceutical products comprise from 30 to 50 percent of a poison center's call volume and account for 39 percent of the reported poisonings to the National Data Collection System of the American Association of Poison Control Centers.

Medications are frequently involved in accidental poisonings in children, since attractive colors of capsules, sugar coating of tablets, flavoring agents, and packaging are all too tempting to the curious toddler. In addition, drugs are among the most often abused substances by older persons, resulting in thousands of suicide and overdose attempts each year. Cyclic antidepressants alone account for 37 percent of all poisoning admissions to medical intensive care units in the United States. Additionally, in 1984 there were 5,743 reported poisonings in physician's offices, clinics, and hospitals, suggesting that iatrogenic, or physician-induced, poisoning is also a problem of some importance.

The drugs included in this section are those most frequently encountered and responsible for the greatest morbidity and mortality in the United States.

CHAPTER 5 *NARCOTIC ANALGESICS*

The narcotic analgesics (Table 5-1) control pain by depressing the central nervous system, although the specific mechanisms by which this is accomplished are complex and beyond the scope of this book.

TABLE 5-1: NARCOTIC ANALGESICS

GENERIC NAME	BRAND NAME	ONSET (MINS)	PEAK (HRS)	DURATION (HRS)
Morphine	Various brands	20	0.5-1.5	up to 7
Hydromorphone	Dilaudid	15-30	0.5-1.5	4-5
Levorphanol	LevoDromoran	60		4-8
Propoxyphene	Darvon	15-30	1-1.5	4-6
Meperidine	Demerol	10-15	0.5-1	2-4
Codeine	Various brands	15-30	1-1.5	4-6
Methadone	Various brands	10-15	1-2	4-6

Historically, the central effect of decreasing pain and inducing euphoria was known in Asia Minor, where the opium poppy is indigenous, since at least 4000 BC. Morphine and other naturally occurring narcotics are alkaloids isolated from one variety of poppy (*Papaver somniferum*). The alkaloids of opium are of two classes: the benzylisoquinolines such as papaverine, which are muscle relaxants without narcotic analgesic effect, and the phenanthrenes, which are the natural occurring narcotic analgesics such as morphine and codeine. The natural occurring alkaloids can be modified chemically to produce other narcotic analgesics such as heroin, methadone, propoxyphene, meperidine, diphenoxylate, and apomorphine. They can also be modified to produce drugs without narcotic analgesic properties such as dextromethorphan and narcotic antagonists such as naloxone. Pentazocine is another chemically modified analgesic that has been widely abused recently in combination with the antihistamine tripelennamine as a street drug.

Poisoning

The clinical manifestations of narcotic analgesic intoxications can be divided into acute and chronic poisoning.

Acute poisoning. It is difficult to give a range of toxicity for narcotic analgesics, since they vary in potency. Codeine seems to be the most frequently encountered in childhood accidents because of the drug's popularity in aspirin and acetaminophen prescription combinations. Children can show minor signs of toxicity with doses as low as 1 mg/kg of codeine; respiratory depression has occurred at 5 mg/kg. The acute toxic effects of narcotic analgesic overdose are several, but the most important is respiratory depression. The patient usually has depressed sensorium and pinpoint pupils; slow, shallow respiration; cyanosis with weak pulse and muscle twitching; paralytic ileus with occasional spasms of the intestine and biliary tract; and in some cases pulmonary edema. Death, if it occurs, is due to respiratory depression. Some narcotic analgesics such as codeine and meperidine produce less respiratory depression and more muscle twitching. Pupillary dilation may accompany meperidine ingestion. Seizures may occur with codeine, meperidine, apomorphine, and propoxyphene. Dextromethorphan is a narcotic derivative without narcotic analgesic properties but its recent introduction into long-acting over-the-counter antitussive formulations has caused problems worthy of special mention. Children ingesting long-acting preparations of dextromethorphan have developed toxicity including ataxia, tachycardia, urticaria, restlessness, lethargy, nystagmus, and blood pressure elevations. This has been observed with doses over 10 mg/kg of dextromethorphan. Naloxone has been reported to have had only partial success in reversing some of these symptoms.

Chronic poisoning. In chronic poisoning from narcotic analgesics the major findings are pinpoint pupils associated with mood changes. Newborns chronically exposed to a narcotic analgesic, such as when mothers are maintained on methadone, show irritability, temperature changes, poor feeding, and constipation with intermittent diarrhea.

The chronic abuse of depressants such as alcohol, barbiturates, and narcotic analgesics produces tolerance and physical dependence. Tolerance development modifies a drug's action by reducing its effects on certain vital mechanisms such as the cardiovascular and respiratory systems. Because all parts of the central nervous system do not become tolerant at the same rate, the brain as a whole is exposed to larger and larger drug concentrations as tolerance develops.

Continuous uninterrupted exposure of the nervous system to large concentrations of depressant drugs induces the phenomenon of physical dependence, which is a state of latent hyperexcitability, resulting when the drug is withdrawn, called the *abstinence syndrome*. The abstinence syndrome is characterized by (1) autonomic hyperactivity including lacrimation, rhinorrhea, sweating, piloerection (gooseflesh), dilated pupils, elevated blood pressure and pulse, hyperpyrexia, abdominal pain, and diarrhea and (2) behavioral hyperexcitability with anxiety, yawning, tremor, insomnia occasionally followed by palpitations and convulsions, and muscle and joint pains. The morphine abstinence or withdrawal syndrome is distressing but rarely life threatening.

Cross tolerance is the phenomenon in which a drug that will prevent withdrawal symptoms is substituted for the drug to which tolerance has developed. Cross tolerance treatment is used more often for narcotic analgesic addicts, in whom a long-acting narcotic (e.g., methadone), which is absorbed orally, is substituted for a short-acting narcotic (e.g., heroin), which is not absorbed orally.

Treatment

In the treatment of acute narcotic analgesic poisoning the most important measures are to maintain respiration and to treat shock, when it is present, in conjunction with the general measures of eliminating and decreasing absorption of the drug as described in Chapter 2.

Pharmacologic antagonists are also very useful in diminishing the effects of a narcotic analgesic. Nalorphine (Nalline) and levallorphan (Lorfan) have been completely replaced by naloxone (Narcan). Nalorphine and levallorphan may depress breathing further if respiratory depression is not due to a narcotic analgesic. Naloxone, however, is a pure narcotic antagonist that has no other pharmacologic effect than to antagonize the narcotic analgesic. It is therefore the antagonist of choice.

The treatment of the chronically addicted patient or drug addict is a difficult sociopsychological problem. From the toxicologic standpoint, one method is to treat the patient by cross tolerance methods, switching him or her to oral propoxyphene or a long-acting, orally absorbed preparation such as methadone. After methadone treatment is instituted, patients can become chronically addicted to the substitute drug if withdrawal is not accomplished by decreasing the doses of the drug over a 1- or 2-week period. A more recent approach is to use the alpha-agonist clonidine (Catapres) to prevent the withdrawal syndrome.

It is postulated that opiates and alpha-adrenergic stimulants inhibit brain regions such as the locus ceruleus, which may be responsible for opiate withdrawal syndrome and other naturally occurring anxiety states. Doses of 0.005 mg/kg/dose orally 2 times daily for 1 week have been used with success. Once a patient is completely drug free, the nonaddicting narcotic antagonist naltrexone, which blocks the effects of opioids, can be taken 3 times weekly. This is an adjunct to a comprehensive treatment program for relapse prevention. Naltrexone cannot cure addiction by itself, but it is pharmacologically effective for up to 3 days, depending on dose, in antagonizing the effects of impulsive opioid use.

References — Chapter 5

H. N. Bhargava, "Mechanism of Toxicity and Rationale for Use of the Combination of Pentazocine and Pyribenzamine in Morphine-Dependant Subjects." *Clin. Toxicol.* 18:175, 1981.

M. S. Gold, D. E. Redmond, and H. D. Keeber, "Noradrenergic Hyperactivity in Opiate Withdrawal Supported by Clonidine Reversal by Opiate Withdrawal." *Am. J. Psychiatry* 136:100-102, 1979.

L. Hershey, and M. Weinetraub, "Easing Morphine Withdrawal in Children." *Drug Ther.* 10:57, 1980.

H. D. Keeber, *Trexan — A Pharmacologic Adjunct for the Detoxified Opiod Addict.* DuPont Product Information, 1984.

M. H. Seevers, "Psychopharmacological Elements of Drug Dependence." *J.A.M.A.* 206:1263-1266, 1968.

D. E. Statzer, and J. N. Wardell, "Heroin Addiction During Pregnancy." *Am. J. Obst. Gynec.* 113:273-278, 1972.

W. O. Sturner, and J. C. Garriott, "Deaths Involving Propoxyphene." *J.A.M.A.* 223:1125-1130, 1973.

L. D. Vandam, "Analgetic Drugs: The Potent Analgetics." *N. Engl. J. Med.* 286:249-253, 1972.

M. L. Warnock, et al., "Pulmonary Complication of Heroin Intoxication: Aspiration Pneumonia and Diffuse Bronchiectasis." *J.A.M.A.* 219:1051-1053, 1972.

C. V. Wetli, J. H. Davis, and B. D. Blackbourne, "Narcotic Addiction in Dade County, Florida: An Analysis of 100 Consecutive Autopsies." *Arch. Path.* 93:330-343, 1972.

D. J. Young, "Propoxyphene Suicides." *Arch. Intern. Med.* 129:62-66, 1972.

CHAPTER 6 NONNARCOTIC ANALGESICS AND ANTIPYRETICS

Nonnarcotic analgesics such as the salicylates, acetaminophen, and the nonsteroidal anti-inflammatory drugs (NSAIDs) are among the agents most frequently prescribed and recommended, and consequently are found in most home medicine chests. Because most nonnarcotic pain relievers are available to the public without prescription, they have traditionally aroused much concern about both acute and chronic poisoning.

SALICYLATES

Because of the reasons just mentioned and because of their incorporation into flavored children's formulations, salicylates have long been a problem in childhood poisoning. Aspirin (acetylsalicylic acid) was consistently the most reported single substance involved in accidental ingestions from the very first annual tabulations by the National Clearing House for Poison Control Centers until 1974. Since 1974 there has been a significant decrease in the frequency of accidental aspirin poisoning, apparently as a result of mandatory use of child-resistant containers as required by the Poison Prevention and Packaging Act of 1970.

Because of the large number of poisonings reported to be caused by salicylates over the years, much investigation on the toxicity of these agents has been conducted. It is worthwhile to consider the metabolism of salicylates before discussing toxicity and treatment.

Salicylates are rapidly absorbed from the gastrointestinal tract, with two thirds of an ingested therapeutic dose absorbed in 1 hour and peak levels in 2 to 4 hours. In overdose, peak levels may be delayed up to 6 hours. After acute overdose of time-release preparations or enteric-coated tablets, peak blood levels may not occur for as long as 28 hours. These alterations in physiologic effect are due to changes in the nature of the dosage form with regard to disintegration time, dissolution rate, rate of absorption, and passage time through the gastrointestinal tract.

After ingestion, the unionized salicylate easily penetrates the stomach's lipid membranes. Once into the circulation and an alkaline environment, it is ionized and trapped in a poorly diffusing state (see Chap. 2). Progression of the intoxication to an acidemic state worsens the situation, since it promotes movement of the salicylate from the vascular and extracellular fluid into the intracellular space. Excretion of a salicylate can be hastened by maintaining an alkaline blood and urine pH. A high urine pH (above 7.5) facilitates salicylate removal by allowing for tubular excretion as opposed to tubular reabsorption, which occurs in an acid urine.

Poisoning

Acute poisoning. Acute ingestion of more than 300 mg/kg is likely to produce local gastrointestinal irritation, direct stimulation of the central nervous system respiratory center, increased metabolic rate, interference with carbohydrate metabolism, and interference with normal blood coagulation mechanisms. In acute salicylate intoxication there is increased oxygen consumption, as well as carbon dioxide and heat production, resulting in increased respiratory rate, heart rate, and cardiac output. The increased metabolic rate and dehydration may worsen the hyperpyrexia.

The nomogram developed by Done (Fig. 6-1) is helpful in relating serum salicylate concentration and expected severity of intoxication at varying intervals following the ingestion of a single dose. Remember that the serum salicylate level is of no value in assessing clinical severity if the drug has been repeatedly administered. After a single oral dose the relationship of clinical status and serum levels in mg/100 ml is as follows: less than 50, usually not intoxicated; 50 to 80, mild symptoms; 80 to 100, moderate intoxication; 100 to 160, severe; above 160, usually lethal. Actually, if a serum level is obtained from 6 to 60 hours after ingestion, the patient's status can be predicted by the Done nomogram to be mild, moderate, or severe. In mild salicylate intoxication moderate hyperpnea sometimes associated with lethargy can be expected. In moderate and severe intoxication there is severe hyperpnea associated in extreme cases with coma and convulsions.

Chronic poisoning. Chronic salicylism is associated with a much higher mortality than acute salicylate poisoning. Chronic poisoning from salicylates produces weight loss, ringing of the ears (tinnitus), and bleeding dyscrasia especially manifested by upper gastrointestinal bleeding, which in severe cases can be accompanied by gastric ulcer. Mental confusion or disorientation, hyperthermia, tachypnea, decreased level of consciousness, and skin rash may also be present. Hepatic encephalopathy not linked to Reye's syndrome has also been reported as a result of chronic salicylate toxicity. Closely monitor patients who receive high doses of

Figure 6-1. Done nomogram for salicylate poisoning. (From "Salicylate Intoxication" by A. K. Done, *Pediatrics* 26:800-807, 1960. Reprinted with permission.)

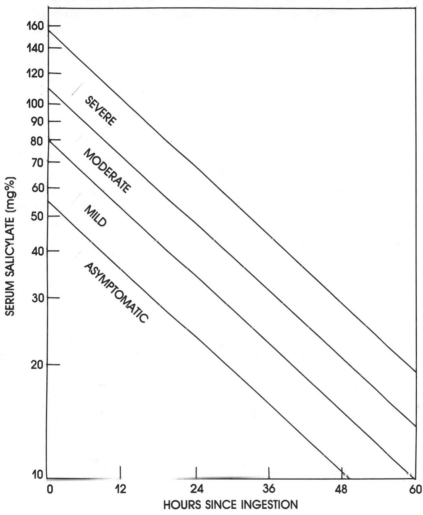

salicylates, particularly children being treated for such conditions as juvenile rheumatoid arthritis, and obtain frequent salicylate blood levels.

Treatment

Design therapy to prevent absorption, to correct fluid deficits, and to reduce tissue levels of the drug. Prevent further absorption by emptying the stomach by lavage or emesis. Administer activated charcoal to adsorb remaining quantities of salicylate in the stomach. Use cathartics, especially if enteric-coated preparations have been ingested (see Chap. 2).

Correcting fluid deficits must ensure the adequacy of the circulating fluid volume and renal perfusion. For initial hydration, administer 5 percent dextrose in 0.45 percent physiologic saline at a rate of 20 ml/kg/hr for the first 1 or 2 hours. In moderate to severe metabolic acidosis, sodium bicarbonate to make an isotonic solution (3.12 g of sodium bicarbonate to 500 ml of 0.45 percent physiologic saline) is added to intravenous fluids.

Adequate urine output must be maintained in addition to alkalinization. The diuretic furosemide at a dose of 1 mg/kg has been recommended as an intravenous additive to obtain a urine flow of 3 to 6 ml/kg/hr.

In severe salicylate poisoning when the patient is in renal insufficiency or fails to respond to more conservative therapy, consider peritoneal dialysis or hemodialysis. Hemodialysis is more effective, but peritoneal dialysis is more generally available.

PARA-AMINOPHENOL DERIVATIVES

Of the para-aminophenol derivatives, known in the nineteenth century as coal tar analgesics (because of their production from coal tar aniline), only acetaminophen has survived into modern drug therapy. Both phenacetin (recently removed from the market) and acetaminophen are closely related in their therapeutic and toxic effects, since acetaminophen (N-acetyl-p-aminophenol) is the major metabolite of phenacetin. The relationship between aniline and the drugs under discussion here is, of course, structural. In addition to being effective analgesics, the para-aminophenol derivatives possess antipyretic properties that reside in the aminobenzene (aniline) structure; however, aniline itself is too toxic for clinical use.

Acetaminophen has replaced phenacetin in all the traditional over-the-counter mixtures. Phenacetin was rarely taken alone, and so acute overdose was complicated by the involvement of other drugs (e.g., aspirin). On the other hand, acetaminophen is often taken alone, and its effects in acute overdose have been well documented, both in England and the United States, where its abuse has grown to considerable proportions.

Poisoning

Acute poisoning. Large single doses of acetaminophen, over 7.5 g, may damage the liver, heart, kidneys, and have been reported to cause respiratory center depression. Liver damage is the most significant problem in acute poisoning with acetaminophen. About 4 percent of a dose of acetaminophen is metabolized by the cytochrome P-450 oxidative pathway to a toxic metabolite. With therapeutic doses of acetaminophen this metabolite is easily conjugated by glutathione and excreted as the nontoxic mercapturate. However, when massive doses of acetaminophen are ingested, glutathione may be depleted in the liver, leaving the toxic metabolite to bind with liver cells and cause cellular death, resulting in hepatic necrosis.

A very significant aspect of overdose is that early signs of poisoning may be minimal, even in cases where death ultimately occurs, since liver damage does not ensue immediately. After an acute overdose vomiting usually occurs in a few hours due to the drug's irritant effects; then come anorexia, nausea, vomiting, and epigastric pain, which may be delayed for 24 hours; transaminase levels become elevated in 2 to 4 days; and jaundice begins in 2 to 6 days. Death may occur at any time from 2 to 7 days. Profound hypoglycemia, metabolic acidosis, acute tubular necrosis, and myocardial necrosis may also complicate severe cases.

Because the major risk in acute intoxication is hepatotoxicity, it is always important to follow hepatic enzyme determinations. Plasma levels of acetaminophen also have predicting value.

Levels of more than 300 micrograms/ml are uniformly associated with hepatic damage, in contrast to lack of toxicity in patients who at 4 hours have levels under 120 micrograms/ml. Patients with levels above 120 micrograms/ml at 4 hours should be treated with N-acetylcysteine.

Chronic poisoning. Phenacetin on a chronic basis has been implicated in producing interstitial nephritis, renal papillary necrosis, and even renal carcinoma. However, phenacetin was often an ingredient of analgesic mixtures and was rarely taken alone. It is thus difficult to determine for certain its long-term adverse effects.

Since 1964 the Food and Drug Administration has required a warning label on phenacetin-containing products stating that the drug "may damage the kidneys when used in large amounts or for a long period of time." In 1984 the drug was removed from the market. The decision was based on the assumption that phenacetin is a common constituent in analgesic remedies taken by subjects who developed interstitial nephritis and papillary necrosis. The difficulty in resolving whether phenacetin alone causes nephritis arises because individuals developing the described renal problems are invariably consumers of many chemicals that make up the broad category of analgesics, supporting the idea of "analgesic" rather than of "phenacetin" nephritis.

In comparing phenacetin with acetaminophen, the latter seems to be the least toxic in long-term administration, although at this point it is purely academic with the removal of phenacetin from the market. Acetaminophen has not been reported to cause liver toxicity even following long-term moderate overdosing. This is most likely due to the fact that glutathione (discussed above) is continually being regenerated in the liver, and levels must fall to below 70 percent of normal of this tripeptide before toxic metabolites of acetaminophen are free to bind with hepatocytes.

Treatment

In the treatment of acute acetaminophen poisoning the emergency measures previously described are always important (see Chap. 2). As in other poisoning episodes, determine as accurately as possible the probable amount ingested, considering the dosage form, concentration, and container volume. Amounts under 150 mg/kg can probably be treated simply by inducing emesis with syrup of ipecac, although treatment based on history alone, particularly following intentional overdoses, is risky. Serum acetaminophen levels are readily available and should be used as a definitive predictor of toxicity. Activated charcoal is also beneficial and should be given in the standard dose of 10 times the weight of the ingested drug. Since acetaminophen plasma levels reach their peak approximately 4 hours after ingestion, induce vomiting and use other methods to prevent absorption before determining plasma level.

Recently, oral N-acetylcysteine (Mucomyst) has been approved by the FDA and widely used as an antidote for acetaminophen poisoning. Other measures such as forced diuresis, hemodialysis, and charcoal hemoperfusion are of little or no value in lowering levels of acetaminophen and in preventing hepatotoxicity. N-acetylcysteine must be used within the first 24 hours after ingestion and is maximally effective if given 10 to 16 hours after ingestion. A loading dose of 140 mg/kg is followed by maintenance oral doses of 70 mg/kg every 4 hours for a total of 18 doses. Intravenous use of N-acetylcysteine is being investigated, and preliminary studies indicate that a 48-hour course of the drug intravenously is more effective in preventing toxicity than either the 72-hour oral method or a shorter 24-hour intravenous course. This consists of the same 140 mg/kg intravenous loading dose and 12 70 mg/kg intravenous maintenance doses at 4-hour intervals. See Chapter 2 for a more detailed discussion of the use of N-acetylcysteine.

PYRAZOLON DERIVATIVES

The pyrazolon class of analgesic agents was originally composed of antipyrine and aminopyrine, but neither compound has survived to any extent today because of high toxicity. The pyrazolon drugs share the anti-inflammatory properties of the salicylates and the analgesic antipyretic effects of the phenacetin/acetaminophen group, but they are more toxic. In popular use today are phenylbutazone (Butazolidin) and oxyphenbutazone (Oxalid), which are close congeners of antipyrine. Also, an analog known as dichloralphenazone is found in the migraine headache remedy, Midrin.

Poisoning

Acute poisoning. The single fatal dose of phenylbutazone and oxyphenbutazone is 5 to 30 g. Fatalities from acute poisoning are rare. However, in large doses pyrazolons stimulate the central nervous system and cause gastrointestinal irritation including nausea, vomiting, epigastric pain, and ulceration. Other reported symptoms from cases of acute poisoning include renal injury including proteinuria, hematuria, water and sodium retention, and even acute nephritis and anuria; hepatic injury; salicylatelike effects such as stimulation of the respiratory center, respiratory alkalosis, metabolic acidosis, tinnitus, and hearing loss; and lethargy, stupor, ataxia, coma, and convulsions.

Chronic poisoning. Therapeutic doses of the pyrazolon drugs may cause moderately toxic reactions such as nausea, vomiting, epigastric discomfort, and skin rash in as many as 50 percent of patients taking some of the least toxic agents such as phenylbutazone. Severe manifestations with prolonged therapeutic use of the pyrazolon group occur in about 5 percent of patients and include hypersensitivity reactions of the serum sickness type, ulcerative stomatitis, hepatitis, nephritis, aplastic anemia, leukopenia, agranulocytosis, and thrombocytopenia.

Treatment

In acute overdose, undertake prevention of absorption by inducing emesis with syrup of ipecac, followed by administering activated charcoal. Give cathartics to speed elimination of unabsorbed drug from the gastrointestinal tract. Ensure adequate hydration with intravenous fluids along with urine output. It has been suggested that, similar to salicylates, an alkaline urinary pH enhances excretion; however, it has not been demonstrated in clinical trials. There is no specific antidote.

Chronic therapeutic use of these drugs should never be without close medical supervision, including laboratory blood work on a weekly basis to avoid serious toxic reactions.

The known factors affecting the incidence of toxic reactions in therapy are age, weight, dosage, duration of therapy, existence of concomitant disease, and concurrent potent chemotherapy. All allergic reactions require prompt and permanent withdrawal of this class of drugs.

NONSTEROIDAL ANTI-INFLAMMATORY DRUGS

The term *nonsteroidal anti-inflammatory drugs* (NSAID) has come by convention to include nonaspirin, nonacetaminophen drugs such as indomethacin (Indocin) and sulindac (Clinoril), which are structurally related; the fenamates, e.g., mefanamic acid (Ponstel); tolmetin (Tolectin) and zomepirac (Zomax); the popular propionic acid derivatives, e.g. ibuprofen (Motrin and Advil) and naproxen (Naprosyn); and piroxicam (Feldene). Several important parameters are shown for these agents in Table 6-1. Most of these drugs share at least something in common with the salicylates. Many of them are better tolerated than salicylates in long-term administration. Nonetheless, they are beginning to demonstrate their toxicity in overdose following wide use in the general population.

Poisoning

Acute poisoning. Most of the symptoms following small overdoses of the NSAIDs are mild and primarily affect the central nervous system and gastrointestinal tract, causing drowsiness, nausea, vomiting, and epigastric pain. More serious reactions such as hypotension, bradycardia, and apnea have been reported but are less frequent. It appears that adults tolerate single acute overdoses much better than children, similar to aspirin overdose. Ingestions of less than 100 mg/kg by history of ibuprofen in

TABLE 6-1: NONSTEROIDAL ANTI-INFLAMMATORY DRUGS

GENERIC NAME	BRAND NAME	ONSET (HRS)	PEAK (HRS)	DURATION (HRS)
Ibuprofen	Motrin	0.5	1-2	4-6
Fenoprofen	Nalfon	Rapid	1-2	
Naproxen	Naprosyn	1	2-4	up to 7
Sulindac	Clinoril	Rapid	1-2	
Indomethacin	Indocin	0.5	2	4-6
Tolmetin	Tolectin	Rapid	0.5-1	
Mefanamic acid	Ponstel	Rapid	2-4	
Piroxicam	Feldene	1	3-5	48-72

children have not been associated with toxicity. Children ingesting 300 mg/kg or more are at risk of developing more serious symptoms described above and should be managed in an emergency facility. Toxic doses for other NSAIDs are less well studied and insufficient data are available to provide ranges of toxicity. As a general rule, slight excesses of the therapeutic dose for these drugs seem to be well tolerated in children and even moderate overdoses are tolerated by adults.

Chronic poisoning. Nephrotic syndrome with acute interstitial nephritis has been reported following therapeutic long-term use (several weeks or longer) of fenoprofen. Cholestatic jaundice with sulindac and diflunisal has been reported. Zomepirac and tolmetin have been associated with a high incidence of anaphylactoid reactions following both acute and chronic use. With zomepiric, thousands of reported reactions have ranged from mild rash to severe anaphylaxis, including at least five

Treatment

Modest overdoses of the NSAIDs are well tolerated by both children and adults. Ingestions of less than 100 mg/kg by history of ibuprofen have not been associated with toxicity and therefore require no treatment. Doses in excess of 100 mg/kg may be treated with emesis, activated charcoal, and cathartics. Additional treatment is supportive and specific symptoms are treated as they arise. Until more is known about other nonsteroidal anti-inflammatory drugs, it seems prudent to induce emesis when two to three times the maximum therapeutic dose is exceeded, and to treat specific symptoms conservatively.
fatalities.

References — Chapter 6

A. K. Done, "Salicylate Intoxication." *Pediatrics* 26:800-807, 1960.

R. Goulding, "Acetaminophen Poisoning." *Pediatrics* 52:6, December 1973.

D. R. Laurence, *Clinical Pharmacology*, 4th ed. (London: Longman, 1973).

R. P. Lofgren, "Fenoprofen Induced Acute Interstitial Nephritis Presenting with Nephrotic Syndrome." *Minn. Med.* 64:287-290, 1981.

A. W. Pierce, "Salicylate Poisoning." *Pediatrics* 54:342-346, 1974.

L. Prescott, et al., "Plasma-Paracetamol Half Life and Hepatic Necrosis in Patients with Paracetamol Overdosage." *Lancet* 1:519, 1971.

A. Proudfoot, et al., "Acute Paracetamol Poisoning." *Br. Med. J.* 3:557, 1970.

S. J. Ratner, "Zomepirac and Renal Failure." *Ann. Intern. Med.* 96:793-794, 1982.

H. C. Rossi, and D. E. Knapp, "Tolmetin Induced Anaphylactoid Reactions." *N. Engl. J. Med.* 307:499-500, 1982.

E. Sutton, and L. F. Soyka, "How Safe is Acetaminophen?" *Clin. Pediat.* 12:12, 692-696, 1976.

CHAPTER 7

STIMULANTS, HALLUCINOGENS, AND DRUGS OF ABUSE

This chapter will discuss stimulant drugs, which are mostly sympathomimetic amines, the substituted amphetamines (hallucinogenic amphetamines), "classical" hallucinogenic drugs, cocaine and phencyclidine (PCP). It has become difficult in recent times to use such labels as "stimulant" or "hallucinogen," particularly with the popularity of the substituted amphetamines. Since many of the drugs discussed in this chapter have no accepted FDA-approved use it is difficult to sort out and quantitate clinical effects in relationship to dose. Numerous reports in the literature regarding the hallucinogenic or psychic effect of these "designer" drugs are not in fact borne out by research, but are recounts of individual experimentation and overdose cases.

One major difference between stimulant and hallucinogenic drugs is in dose response: it takes a larger dose of a stimulant than of a hallucinogenic drug to stimulate the central nervous system. Thus, the small pharmacologic effect of the stimulants on the brain tends to induce psychotoxic reaction less often than does the hallucinogenic effect.

STIMULANTS

Stimulant drugs may be sympathomimetic amines such as epinephrine, ephedrine, and related drugs that are widely used for their vasoconstrictor and bronchodilator effects (Table 7-1). Amphetamine is also a sympathomimetic drug once used as an anorectic and mood elevator and, controversially, in the treatment of hyperactive children alone or with methylphenidate. Amphetamine analogs have replaced amphetamine for appetite suppression. These are adrenergic amines such as diethylpropion (Tenuate) and benzphetamine (Didrex) (Table 7-2).

TABLE 7-1: SYMPATHOMIMETIC AGENTS

PARENTERAL:	ONSET (MINS)	DURATION (HRS)
Epinephrine (various brands)	immediate 5	less than 1
ORAL:		
Ephedrine (component of numerous asthma and over-the-counter preparations)	15-60	3-5
Phenylephrine (Neosynephrine)	15-30	2-4
Phenylpropanolamine (over-the-counter diet preparation, decongestant, Dexatrim-15, Propagest)	15-30	3
Pseudoephedrine (Sudafed)	15-30	4-8
Terbutaline (Brethine)	30	4-8
TOPICAL:		
Naphazoline (Privine)	1-5	3-6
Oxymetazoline (Afrin, Duration)	1-5	6-12
Tetrahydrozoline (Tyzine nasal decongestant, Visine ophthalmic solution)	1-5	3-6
Xylometazoline (Otrivin)	1-5	6-12
INHALATION:		
Isoetharine (Bronkosol)	1	1-3
Metaproterenol (Alupent)	1-5	3-4
Albuterol (Proventil)	within 30	4-6

Caffeine is a popular central nervous system stimulant employed in many over-the-counter stimulant and "street" drugs. Chemically it is an xanthine derivative, structurally different from the sympathomimetic amines and related to theophylline and theobromine (see xanthine derivatives, Chap. 10).

TABLE 7-2: AMPHETAMINE ANALOGS

DRUG	BRAND EXAMPLE
Amphetamine	Generic only
Benzphetamine	Didrex
Dextroamphetamine	Dexedrine
Diethylpropion	Tenuate
Methamphetamine	Desoxyn
Phendimetrazine	Bontril PDM
Phenmetrazine	Preludin
Phentermine	Fastin

Poisoning

The principal manifestations of poisoning from these drugs are central nervous system stimulation and cardiovascular changes including blood pressure elevation. Therapeutically the sympathomimetic amines have been used for their mood-elevating properties, which is also the reason for psychological addiction; that is, addicts seek the reward of their mood elevation effects. However, there is no true physical dependence as manifest by definite physical abstinence syndrome.

Acute poisoning. Acute poisoning from sympathomimetic amines produces central nervous system stimulation associated with nervousness, irritability, nausea, vomiting, and, in extreme cases, convulsions and hallucinations. Like all sympathomimetic amines, stimulants also produce pupillary dilation, which is associated with blurred vision, vasoconstriction, and tachycardia, resulting in hypertension that may be followed by hypotension and diarrhea. Hypertension-induced reflex bradycardia can also occur. Caffeine is a naturally occurring alkaloid that is rarely associated with serious adverse reactions or fatalities. Relatively small doses of caffeine produce such unpleasant effects, such as gastritis and jitteriness, that this probably accounts for the lack of fatalities. Overdose has produced cardiac stimulation resulting in a variety of arrhythmias. From both the sympathomimetic amines and caffeine the tachycardia may progress very rarely to ventricular arrhythmia and myocardial infarction. Intracerebral hemorrhage has been reported to occur with pseudoephedrine, even while the patient remains normotensive, leading to the suggestion that this drug can cause a direct cerebral vasculitic effect. When these compounds are injected, the local vasoconstriction produced may result in necrosis and sloughing of skin and subcutaneous tissue.

Chronic poisoning. The chronic use of the sympathomimetic amines results in a phenomenon called *primary psychological dependence*. In other words, no physical withdrawal symptoms occur, but the person becomes psychologically addicted to the drug's effect. Prolonged nasal use of these drugs results in a local rebound vascular effect in which the nose becomes congested. Chronically addicted patients have dilated pupils and are usually irritable and unstable, and with larger doses these effects may progress to increasing tension, anxiety, and eventually to hallucinations and psychosis.

It is fairly well accepted that a certain degree of tolerance and psychic dependence develops to the prolonged use of caffeine-containing beverages. Sudden withdrawal from caffeine has been reported to cause headaches that are relieved by consuming caffeine.

Treatment

Emesis is not indicated if the patient is seen at or beyond the time of onset of activity for sympathomimetic drugs (Table 7-1). If performed at all, it should immediately follow ingestion due to the potential for seizures, aggravation of high blood pressure, and cardiovascular complications. Gastric lavage followed by activated charcoal may be the best alternative. Hyperactivity may be controlled with diazepam. Seizures should be managed with diazepam, phenytoin, or phynobarbital, and as a last resort, neuromuscular blocking agents. When a neuromuscular blocking agent, such as pancuronium bromide is used, the patient is mechanically ventilated and the EEG is monitored to ensure cessation of cerebral seizure activity. Sodium nitroprusside should be considered in the event of hypertensive emergencies. Beta blockers have been suggested for the treatment of pseudoephedrine-induced tachyarrhythmias and hypertension. Their use may lead to unopposed peripheral alpha stimulation (vasoconstriction) with resulting exacerbation of hypertension. Labetalol (Trandate, Normodyne) has been suggested as an alternative to beta blockers when treating hypertension since it effectively blocks both beta and alpha receptors.

SUBSTITUTED AMPHETAMINES

Also referred to as "hallucinogenic amphetamines," these drugs belong to the amphetamine group, but their chemical structure has been altered, creating a substance with hallucinogenic properties. However, the effects of these chemicals may vary widely from what is meant by hallucinogenic when talking about other drugs, such as LSD. The newer substances on the street, particularly MDMA, are claimed to induce a lesser degree of perceptual disturbances than the "true" hallucinogens, making them preferable as recreational drugs.

The alphabet soup of these drugs includes:

- DMA (2,5-dimethoxyamphetamine);
- DOB (4-bromo-dimethoxyamphetamine);
- DOET (4-ethyl-dimethoxyamphetamine);
- DOM of "STP" fame (2,5-dimethoxy-4-methylamphetamine);
- MDA (3,4-methylenedioxyamphetamine), first synthesized in 1910 and probably the simplest of these substituted compounds;
- MDMA (3,4-methylenedioxymethamphetamine), the substance of choice for most users in the 1980s, even though this drug was first synthesized in 1914 by Merck Co. as an appetite suppressant but never marketed;
- MMDA (3-methoxy-4,5-methylenedioxyamphetamine);
- DMMDA (2,5-dimethoxy-methlenedioxyamphetamine);
- PMA (para-methoxyamphetamine); and
- TMA (3,4,5-trimethoxyamphetamine).

Poisoning

Acute poisoning. Excitement, agitation, anorexia, and nystagmus are very common, early signs following use of the substituted amphetamines. These may be accompanied by numerous other complaints and symptoms, such as nausea, vomiting, diarrhea, and diaphoresis. An increase in respiratory rate with hypertension and tachycardia is frequently observed in mildly affected patients. Dilated pupils are almost always present. In severe poisoning, cardiac arrhythmias and cardiovascular collapse leading to shock may occur. Delirium, seizures, and coma may be seen. In substantial overdoses a whole range of muscle spasm may occur leading to rhabdomyolysis, myoglobinemia, and myoglobinuria.

Chronic poisoning. Prolonged use of the substituted amphetamines leads to many of the problems seen with the traditional amphetamines and hallucinogens. Antisocial behavior, emotional instability, paranoia, and other inappropriate behavior is found in individuals who regularly use these substances.

Treatment

Agitation, hallucinations, and excitement are treated with diazepam, either orally or intravenously. The major tranquilizers, such as the phenothiazines and butyrophenones are not generally recommended to control minor agitation and excitement, because of undesirable side effects with these medications. However, heloperidol (Haldol) has been recommended as possibly effective in the treatment of severe poisoning from hallucinogenic amphetamines. Seizures should be controlled with diazepam, phenytoin, or phenobarbital. If these drugs are not effective, the patient must be paralyzed with pancuronium with EEG monitoring and mechanical ventilation. Supraventricular cardiac arrhythmias are not treated with medication unless there is hemodynamic instability, such as hypotension or poor perfusion. Ventricular arrhythmias are treated with lidocaine, bretylium tosylate, phenytoin, or propranolol depending on the circumstances and condition of the patient. Hypotension is initially treated with intravenous fluids and positioning, and as a last resort dopamine or norepinephrine. Late developing rhabdomyolysis and myoglobinuria may be treated with alkaline diuresis.

COCAINE

Cocaine is found in the leaves of the plant Erythroxylon coca and was first isolated in 1860. It is similar to the amphetamines in pharmacologic activity but differs somewhat chemically. The pharmaceutical grade cocaine salts are white, crystalline powders resembling snow, hence its street name. In addition to its local anesthetic properties, it is a powerful central nervous system stimulant.

Cocaine abuse continues as a persistent problem in the United States. Newer, cheaper, street forms of the free base (cocaine sulfate), known by "crack" and other names, may appear as yellow, wax-like chunks or flakes. The yellow discoloration is presumably due to adulterants. The various salts and physical forms of cocaine may be "snorted" intranasally, injected, or smoked with tobacco or marijuana.

Cocaine is a local anesthetic and vasoconstrictor but its toxicity is mainly due to its effect on the central nervous system and cardiovascular systems with a resulting biphasic patterns of extreme excitation followed by depression. Most cocaine fatalities occur acutely and are caused by respiratory depression and/or persistent hypotension. Sudden, fatal, cardiac dysrhythmia has been reported with use of free base cocaine. Free basing seems to present an increased risk of cardiac death from cocaine. Intranasal use of the hydrochloride salt causes local vasoconstriction which limits and delays absorption of cocaine. Since the free base is more stable to destruction by heat than the hydrochloride salt, it can be smoked and smoking offers no such protection.

Poisoning

Acute poisoning. Following cocaine use, mental changes vary from euphoria, excitement, restlessness, and anxiety to delirium and acute paranoid psychosis. At first the increased motor activity is well coordinated but as lower motor centers are affected, tremulousness, hyperreflexia, and fasciculations become apparent. Tonic-clonic seizures can occur, frequently followed by central nervous system depression. Nausea and vomiting may occur due to stimulation of the brain. Severe respiratory and metabolic acidosis have been seen as a result of seizure activity. Most respiratory effects are due to medullary stimulation or depression. At first an increase in rate and depth of respiration occurs followed by rapid shallow breathing that may deteriorate to Cheyne-Stokes pattern in larger doses. Respiratory arrest may follow. Pulmonary edema has been reported. Small doses of cocaine cause an increase in heart rate and blood pressure. A reflex bradycardia may result if hypertension is significant. With larger doses hypotension precedes tachyarrhythmias due to the loss of sympathetic tone. Sinus tachycardia is the most frequent finding followed by reports of premature ventricular contractions (PVCs), bigeminy, accelerated ventricular arrhythmias, and ventricular fibrillation. Large intravenous doses can result in immediate death from cardiac failure due to direct myocardial toxicity. Hyperthermia can result due to increased muscular activity, vasoconstriction, and perhaps a direct effect on the hypothalamus. Animal studies show that hyperthermia may be the most important factor contributing to cocaine death.

Chronic poisoning. Chronic, heavy use of cocaine may cause sleeplessness, anorexia, restlessness, paranoia, violent outbursts, unrelieved fatigue, lapses in attention, inability to concentrate, sexual impotency, severe depression, and toxic psychosis. Perceptual alterations or hallucinations involving touch, vision, geometric patterns, smell, hearing, and taste may occur after several months of recreational cocaine use and during times of increased usage.

Treatment

Most mild intoxications resulting in sinus tachycardia and mildly elevated blood pressure can be treated with supportive care. Seizures are treated with diazepam, phenytoin, or phenobarbital. Hypotension should initially be treated by putting the patient in a Trendelenburg position and administering intravenous fluids. If the patient is unresponsive to these measures administer dopamine (Intropin) or levarterenol (Levophed). Hypertension is usually transient and ordinarily does not require treatment. Cardiac arrhythmias have been treated with propranolol, lidocaine, or phenytoin. Verapamil (Calan, Isoptin) and other calcium channel blockers have been suggested, but not much clinical experience exists to support the effectiveness of these agents in the management of cocaine overdose. Hyperthermia is treated with usual conservative methods, placing the patient in a cool room, decreasing physical activity, sponging with water, and use of a hypothermic blanket. Hyperthermia can plan an important role in causing cocaine induced deaths. At the present time the use of drugs to control hyperthermia is not supported by enough evidence. To control psychosis or anxiety the patient should be placed in a dark and quiet area and treated in a calm reassuring manner. Diazepam, orally or intravenously, may be helpful.

HALLUCINOGENS

The hallucinogens include such strong sympathomimetic drugs as lysergic acid diethylamide (LSD), marijuana, and so forth. None produces physical dependence as do the depressants such as alcohol, barbiturates, and narcotic analgesics, but like the stimulants they produce primary psychological dependence. All are central nervous system stimulants, but the effect of a given dose is greater than in the case of stimulants such as epinephrine. With the hallucinogens, distortion occurs as an early manifestation in the dose-response curve.

The more truly hallucinogenic drugs are mostly amphetamine congeners such as LSD. LSD is an antiserotonin-modified ergot alkaloid with an unusual hallucinogenic potency. Morning glory seeds contain amides of lysergic acid. Peyote, from a species of cactus, is also hallucinogenic, since it contains mescaline, an epinephrine like compound. Antiserotonin tryptamine derivatives such as psilocybin, which comes from the mushroom *Psilocybe mexicana*, and dimethyltryptamine (DMT) are also hallucinogenic.

Marijuana or hashish is frequently grouped with the stimulant mild hallucinogenic drugs because it induces a dreamy state, with a marked tendency to fantasize and accept suggestions. Marijuana comes from the hemp plant *Cannabis sativa* whose active principle is tetrahydrocannabinol (THC), present in the resin concentrated in the flowering tips. The collected concentrated resin is known as hashish. Actually, marijuana, hashish, or tetrahydrocannabinol produces the dream state not as a stimulant drug but as a sedative or hypnotic by decreasing inhibitions, similar to the euphoric state induced by alcohol. Marijuana even produces a mild state of hyperexcitability on withdrawal suggestive of the mild abstinence syndrome expected from a sedative or hypnotic and not from a stimulant or hallucinogen.

Poisoning

Acute poisoning. The patient poisoned by a hallucinogen will have acute problems similar to those of the patient intoxicated with a stimulant drug. Manifestations are hyperirritability, hypertension, mydriasis, tremors, and increased deep tendon reflexes, but the anxiety and excitation are more severe and frequently lead to a psychotic state.

Chronic poisoning. The chronic use of hallucinogens also results in problems similar to those in stimulant overuse, but the psychopathic state is chronic. With LSD and similar drugs, flashbacks (sudden recurrences of perceptual distortion experienced during the drug experience) occur.

Treatment

Emergency measures to decrease the absorption of hallucinogens through either oral or parenteral ports of entry are those described in Chapter 2.

Acute anxiety is best managed with oral or intravenous diazepam. Emesis is usually not effective because most adult patients are not seen in the emergency department until long after the initial administration of the drug. However, children occasionally accidentally ingest hallucinogenic substances belonging to their parents or adults with custody. If seen early in an emergency department, emesis and charcoal administration may be effective measures.

The major tranquilizers of the phenothiazine group, such as chlorpromazine (Thorazine), are reported by some to be useful antidotes to calm hallucinogen-induced anxiety states. However, these tranquilizers may be dangerous in poisonings with some stimulant and hallucinogenic drugs (e.g., DMT) and also fail to calm drug-induced anxiety due to parasympatholytic drugs such as atropine and scopolamine, which can be used to "cut" certain of the stimulants and hallucinogens. Of course, blood pressure must be monitored in patients poisoned by hallucinogens. If blood pressure is significantly elevated, the patient must receive anti-hypertensive drugs to prevent hypertensive bleeding.

PHENCYCLIDINE

Phencyclidine (PCP) is an illicit drug whose use has been prevalent for some time. Not only is PCP use common in adults, but numerous reports of inadvertent or accidental ingestion or inhalation in infants and toddlers exist. Phencyclidine is a potent sympathomimetic and hallucinogenic anesthetic agent that is structurally related to the legitimate anesthetic ketamine.

Poisoning

Acute poisoning. Phencyclidine poisoning has been described in stages that seem to be clinically useful. Stage I is a low-level overdose where the patient is conscious although very disoriented and possibly violent or self-destructive. Stage II is a state of moderate dose where the patient is unconscious but stable. Stage III is a state of severe intoxication that may involve adrenergic crisis, seizures, and respiratory failure.

PCP is similar to ketamine in producing anesthesia. In stage I it usually produces agitation, ataxia, hyperreflexia, and excitation with marked paranoid behavior, frequently self-destructive. Horizontal and vertical nystagmus, flushing, seizures, muscle rigidity, respiratory depression, and coma with the eyes open are common diagnostic clues. Delayed toxicity may be seen for 3 or 4 days following a major overdose, possibly due to distribution into the lipid tissues. Tachycardia and hypertension may be noted. Although extremely rare, massive fatal intracranial hemorrhage (possibly due to the drug's acute hypertensive effect) in the absence of trauma has been reported in one patient. Noncardiogenic pulmonary edema was also noted at the time of the bleed. Rhabdomyolysis, myoglobinuria, acute uric acid nephropathy, and associated acute renal failure have been reported following PCP intoxication.

Chronic poisoning. Chronic users of PCP develop tolerance to its effects and can consume much larger doses in a 24-hour period. Some users have complained of persistent cognitive and memory problems. Speech difficulties, including stuttering and poor articulation, may occur and have persisted. Depression, anxiety, weight loss, and violent or self-destructive behavior are frequent with chronic use; purposeful activity is almost impossible. Paranoid and violent behavior with auditory hallucinations appear, and the schizophrenic state may last for weeks and may recur without reuse of the drug. Some patients have recovered completely, while others appear to display a sustained chronic brain syndrome.

Treatment

In an acute poisoning, establish respiration and refer to Chapter 2 for methods of preventing absorption with charcoal and cathartics. Ipecac is contraindicated due to the likelihood of seizures. Gastric lavage and charcoal may be useful to remove the drug even if smoked or snorted, since PCP is secreted into the stomach. Intravenous diazepam may be used in patients experiencing seizures.

Administering a diuretic such as furosemide in combination with urine acidification increases the urinary excretion of PCP. Although acidification significantly increases the renal clearance of PCP, the total amount of drug removed is minimal because of the large volume of PCP distribution. Acidification can precipitate acute renal failure in patients with rhabdomyolysis and should be avoided in this setting. Ascorbic acid may be administered every 6 hours intravenously up to 8 g/day to acidify the blood. Urine pH should return to a pH of 4.5 to 5.5. Treat rhabdomyolysis and associated myoglobinuria with intravenous fluids and sodium bicarbonate. Minimize all sensory stimuli such as noise, light, and touch. Treat symptomatic hypertensive crisis with intravenous nitroprusside or phentolamine. Significant reduction of psychomimetic effects from bad "trips" can be achieved by providing a quiet and nonthreatening environment. Protect the agitated and excited patient from self-inflicted injury. Of course, it may be difficult to tell PCP psychosis from non-PCP psychosis. Behaviorial problems can be managed with intravenous diazepam, which should be administered as a first means of treatment. Manage severe behavioral problems with haloperidol, 2 to 5 mg intramuscularly every 1 to 8 hours up to 100 mg/day in an adult. Haloperidol at a dose of 5 to 10 mg has been reported to improve many phencyclidine-induced symptoms characteristic of schizophrenia (e.g., auditory hallucinations, bizarre delusions, and disorganized thinking).

References — Chapter 7

Editorial, "Amphetamines." *N. Z. Med. J.* 75:160, 1972.

J. S. Bowen, et al., "Diffuse Vascular Spasm Associated with 4-bromo-2, 5-dimethoxyamphetamine Ingestion." *J.A.M.A.* 249:1477-1479, 1983.

A. J. Dietz, "Amphetamine-Like Reactions to Phenylpropanolamine." *J.A.M.A.* 245:601, 1981.

B. H. Fookes, "Psychosis after LSD." *Lancet* 1:1074-1075, 1972.

M. Gabel, "Treatment of Ingestion of LSD." *J. Pediatr.* 81:634, 1972.

L. M. Haddad, and J. F. Winchester (ed.), *Clinical Management of Poisoning and Drug Overdose*, "Cocaine," Philadelphia: W.B. Saunders, 1983, pp. 443-447.

B. M. Ianzito, B. Liskow, and M. A. Steward, "Reaction to LSD in a 2-Year-Old Child." *J. Pediatr.* 80:643-645, 1972.

C. Jackson, A. Hart, and M. D. Robinson, "Fatal Intracranial Hemorrhage Associated with Phenylpropanolamine, Pentazocine, and Triplennamine Overdose," *J. Emerg. Med.* 3:127-132, 1985.

E. C. Klatt, et al., "Misrepresentation of Stimulant Street Drugs: A Decade of Experience in an Analysis Program." *Clin. Toxicol.*, 24:441-450, 1986.

A. Klepfisz, and J. Racy, "Homicide and LSD." *J.A.M.A.* 223:429-430, 1973.

H. Kolansky, and W. T. Moore, "Effect of Marihuana on Adolescents and Young Adults." *J.A.M.A.* 216:486-492, 1971.

C. M. Liberman, and B. W. Lieberman, "Marihuana: A Medical Review." *N. Engl. J. Med.* 284:88-91, 1971.

G. M. Marquardt, V. Distephano, and L. L. Ling, "Pharmacological and Toxicological Effects of B-3, 4-methylenedioxyamphetamine Isomers." *Toxicol. Appl. Pharmacol.* 45:675-683, 1978.

G. G. Nathas, "Cannabis Sativa: The Deceptive Weed." *N. Y. J. Med.* 72:856-868, 1972.

D. Reed, R. H. Cravey, and P. R. Sedgwick, "A Fatal Case Involving Methylenedioxyamphetamine." *Clin. Toxicol.* 5:3-6, 1972.

M. H. Seevers, "Psychopharmacological Elements of Drug Dependence." *J.A.M.A.* 206:1263-1266, 1968.

D. E. Smith, and C. Mehl, "An Analysis of Marijuana Toxicity." *Clin. Toxicol.* 3:101-116, 1970.

J. L. Sullivan, "Caffeine Poisoning in an Infant." *J. Pediatr.* 90:1022-1023, 1977.

B. H. Waters, and Y. D. LaPierre, "Secondary Mania with Sympathomimetic Drug Use." *Am. J. Psychol.* 138:837-841, 1981.

G. E. Woody, "Visual Disturbances Experienced by Hallucinogenic Drug Abusers While Driving." *Am. J. Psychiatry.* 127:431-436, 1970.

E. G. Zalis, G. D. Lundberg, and R. A. Knutson, "The Pathophysiology of Acute Amphetamine Poisoning with Pathologic Correlation." *J. Pharmacol. Exp. Ther.* 158:115-127, 1967.

CHAPTER 8

DEPRESSANTS: BARBITURATES AND ALCOHOL

The central nervous system depressants include narcotic analgesics (see Chap. 5), barbiturates (Table 8-1), and alcohol. All three reduce mental and physical functions. Chronic abuse of the depressants is associated with tolerance and physical dependence (see Chap. 5).

BARBITURATES

Barbiturates are the major drugs used in suicide. All barbiturates are derivatives of barbituric acid with different side chains. In general, barbiturates with long side chains (e.g., secobarbital) have a short duration of action; those with short side chains (e.g., phenobarbital) have a long duration of action (Table 8-1).

Long-acting barbiturates are less bound to plasma protein than are the short-acting agents. The pK of a drug is the pH at which the ionized and nonionized forms of an acid or base are equal in concentration. All barbiturates are weak organic acids but have somewhat different pKs, which determines to an extent their specific duration of action. Usually, short-acting barbiturates have a pK that makes them mostly nonionized at the physiologic pH (secobarbital is 2 percent ionized) and thus are more lipid soluble and excreted in smaller amounts by the kidney and by dialysis. Long-acting compounds have a pK that allows them to be ionized mostly at the physiologic pH (phenobarbital is 95 percent ionized) and thus are more water soluble and excreted in larger amounts by the kidney and by dialysis.

All barbiturates undergo biotransformation in the liver, but the short-acting drugs depend entirely on hepatic degradation. Only two thirds or less of the long-acting barbituates are degraded by the liver; the rest is excreted.

Poisoning

Acute poisoning. The major problem with all sedative and hypnotic

TABLE 8-1: BARBITURATES

GENERIC NAME	BRAND NAME	ONSET (MINS)	PEAK (HRS)
Phenobarbital	Various brands	60 or longer	10-12
Mephobarbital	Mebaral	60 or longer	10-12
Amobarbital	Amytal	45-60	6-8
Butabarbital	Butisol	45-60	6-8
Secobarbital	Seconal	10-15	3-4
Pentobarbital	Nembutal	10-15	3-4

drugs is central nervous system depression to the point of coma. Sleepiness and confusion are the first manifestations, followed by more severe coma (grades 0 to 4) depending on the size of the dose. Patients in grade 0 coma are arousable; patients in grade 1 are nonarousable but responsive to pain; in grade 2, unresponsive to pain but reflexes are intact; in grade 3, have no deep tendon reflex but vital signs are stable; in grade 4, have respiratory or circulatory instability. Rapid intravenous injection of any barbiturate may also cause immediate laryngospasm, hypotension, and severe respiratory depression. Patients tolerate higher blood barbiturate levels with long-acting barbiturates than with short-acting compounds. For example, 3 mg/100 ml is a high level for secobarbital but not for phenobarbital; 8 mg/100 ml would be a high level for phenobarbital.

Chronic poisoning. The chronic use of barbiturates, like use of other depressants such as alcohol and narcotic analgesics, can produce tolerance and physical addiction with a well-defined abstinence syndrome. In rapid withdrawal from prolonged continuous use, the abstinence syndrome is usually characterized by anxiety, insomnia, muscular twitching, tremors, and even convulsions.

Treatment

Treatment requires the emergency measures described in Chapter 2. In the presence of laryngospasm, insert an endotracheal tube, for which a tracheotomy may be necessary. Respiratory and cardiac arrest are always possibilities during intubation. Some severely poisoned patients in grade 4 coma may also require treatment for shock.

Analeptic drugs such as pentylenetetrazol and methylphenidate have been used in the past but are now clearly contraindicated, since they have been shown to worsen the condition and increase mortality in overdosed patients. Forced diuresis with alkalization of the urine and dialysis are of help in the treatment of patients poisoned by long-acting barbiturates because they are more water soluble and less plasma protein bound than short-acting barbiturates.

The treatment of chronic barbiturate addiction is often a major psychosocial problem. Pharmacologically, the abstinence syndrome is like the narcotic analgesic withdrawal syndrome, a state of central nervous system hyperexcitability characterized by delirium, hallucinations, tremors, hyperthermia, and convulsions. Barbiturate withdrawal can be intense enough to be life threatening.

ETHYL ALCOHOL

Ethyl alcohol is a short-acting sedative and hypnotic central nervous system depressant. Since the beginning of history almost all fruit juices, plant saps and fibers, honey, and grains have been fermented to produce alcoholic beverages. In addition to ethanol, fermentation also produces congeners or higher alcohols and aldehydes, acids, esters, and ketones, of which the most common are isoamyl alcohol (fusel oil) and ethyl acetate. These are longer-acting depressants than ethyl alcohol and are present both in distilled beverages and in wine. Brandy and wine also contain traces of methyl alcohol from the pectin of grapes.

Alcoholic beverages are short-acting sedatives and hypnotics with peak levels after oral ingestion at 40 minutes and clearing by 8 hours. The fatal dose of ethanol is approximately 6 ml/kg of body weight of 100 percent alcohol or 12 ml/kg of body weight of an alcoholic beverage that is 100 proof.

Poisoning

Acute poisoning. At a blood alcohol level between 50 and 150 mg/100 ml, the patient is delighted and uninhibited. Definitely sluggish reflexes occur at a level of 100 mg/100 ml of blood. A level above 100 mg/100 ml is usually reached by a 75 kg person after three drinks of 100 percent proof alcohol of 1 oz each in less than 1 hour. One ounce of 100 proof alcohol is comparable to one 4-oz glass of wine or 12 oz of beer. At levels of 150 to 300 mg/100 ml the patient is confused and has impaired vision, speech, and muscle coordination. At levels above 300 mg/100 ml there is marked muscular incoordination, blurred vision, slurred speech, stupor, and even coma. Death may follow respiratory arrest. Hypoglycemia, which is worse in children, may occur, together with hypothermia in acute alcohol intoxication. The drunkometer estimates the blood alcohol level by measuring the weight of alcohol in 190 mg of expired carbon dioxide.

Chronic poisoning. The psychosocial problems leading to alcoholism are somewhat similar to those in people addicted to other central nervous system depressants and are not entirely within the scope of this book (see Chap. 5).

Chronic alcoholism may lead to polyneuritis, encephalopathy (Wernicke's encephalopathy), cardiomyopathy (similar to beriberi), fatty degeneration and cirrhosis of the liver, and even psychosis (Korsakoff's psychosis). Folic acid, vitamin B_{12}, and other B complex deficiencies such as beriberi and pellagra as well as iron deficiency anemia may all occur in chronic alcoholics. Sudden withdrawal of alcohol in addicted persons leads to an abstinence syndrome characterized by hyperexcitability, restlessness, agitation, and insomnia that may lead to psychosis (delirium tremens).

Treatment

The emergency treatment of acute alcoholic intoxication requires the basic principles described in Chapter 2. Maintain an airway and supportive respiration. Since alcohol inhibits antidiuretic hormone, administer fluids carefully and with glucose, since hypoglycemia may occur. Dialysis is indicated with blood alcohol levels above 500 mg/100 ml.

The pharmacologic principle in the treatment of the chronic alcoholic is to replace a short-acting sedative such as alcohol with a long-acting sedative such as chlordiazepoxide. Multivitamins are also needed because alcoholic polyneuritis as well as cardiomyopathy and encephalopathy are mostly due to thiamine deficiency. Several other nutritional deficiencies, described previously, also occur in chronic alcoholics.

Disulfiram is used in the treatment of rehabilitated chronic alcoholics. It blocks the metabolism of alcohol by interfering with alcohol dehydrogenase and resulting in accumulation of acetaldehyde, which makes the patient who drinks alcohol very uncomfortable.

OTHER ALCOHOLS

Methyl alcohol is obtained from destructive distillation of wood. It is used as an antifreeze, paint remover, solvent in shellac and varnish, and denaturant of alcohol. Methanol is metabolized by the same enzyme as ethyl alcohol to formic acid, which is extremely toxic, causing optic atrophy and cardiac depression and damaging the liver and kidneys. However, it is metabolized and excreted more slowly than ethyl alcohol. Thus, ethyl alcohol, by depleting the stores of alcohol dehydrogenase, is useful in the treatment of methanol intoxication. Methanol is also dialyzable.

Isopropyl alcohol is used in rubbing alcohol, in cosmetics such as aftershave lotions, and in window cleaning products. It is twice as toxic as ethyl alcohol and not as toxic as methyl alcohol because isopropyl alcohol is metabolized to ethyl alcohol, not to methanol. to ethyl alcohol. Also, approximately 15 percent is converted to acetone. Pulmonary damage may result when the lungs excrete isopropyl alcohol.

Denatured alcohol is ethyl alcohol denatured with certain additives such as small amounts of methyl (5 percent) and, more commonly, of brucine (especially in cosmetics) alkaloid together with tert butyl alcohol. Since ethanol is metabolized faster than methanol, oxidation of this small amount (5 percent) of methanol is inhibited by the large amount of ethanol present in denatured alcohol. The quantity of brucine alkaloid in denatured alcohol is insufficient to cause problems. Thus, the treatment is similar to that for ethanol poisoning.

Ethylene glycol is used in antifreeze and, like methanol, is very toxic. Ethylene glycol is metabolized to oxalic acid and, like methanol, also by alcohol dehydrogenase. Thus in ethylene glycol intoxication, as with methanol intoxication, treatment consists of ethyl alcohol to compete with the enzyme alcohol dehydrogenase to block metabolism to the toxic metabolite oxalic acid.

References — Chapter 8

B. R. Abernathy, et al., "Treatment of Diazepam Withdrawal Syndrome with Propranolol." *Ann. Intern. Med.* 94:354-357, 1981.

H. C. Aquino, and C. D. Leonard, "Ethylene Glycol Poisoning: Report of 3 Cases." *J. Kentucky Med. Assoc.* 70:463:465, 1972.

K. Closs, and C. O. Solberg, "Methanol Poisoning." *J.A.M.A.* 211:497-499, 1970.

E. G. Comstock, "Glutethimide Intoxication." *J.A.M.A.* 215:1668, 1971.

Criteria Committee, National Council on Alcoholism, "Criteria for the Diagnosis of Alcoholism." *Ann. Int. Med.* 77:249-258, 1972.

E. A. Cuttler, et al., "Delayed Cardiopulmonary Arrest after Lomotil Ingestion." *Pediatrics.* 65:157-159, 1980.

M. J. Goldberg, and W. G. Belinger, "Treatment of Phenobarbital Overdose with Activated Charcoal." *J.A.M.A.* 247:2400-2404, 1982.

N. F. Gumpert, "Criteria for the Use of Specific Forms of Therapy for Barbiturate Overdose." *Am. J. Hosp. Pharmocol.* 29:428-433, 1972.

J, Hadden, et al., "Acute Barbiturate Intoxication." *J.A.M.A.* 209:893-900, 1969.

R. D. Hawkins, and H. Kalant, "The Metabolism of Ethanol and Its Metabolic Effect." *Pharmacol. Rev.* 24:67-157, 1972.

R. E. Johnstone, and R. L. Witt, "Respiratory Effects of Alcohol Intoxication." *J.A.M.A.* 222:486, 1972.

A. C. Kennedy, et al., "Successful Treatment of 3 Cases of Very Severe Barbiturate Poisoning." *Lancet* 1:995-997, 1969.

W. S. Lovell, "Breath Tests for Determining Alcohol in the Blood." *Science* 178:264-272, 1972.

H. Mathew, P. Roscoe, and N. Wright, "Acute Poisoning: A Comparison of Hypnotic Drugs." *Practitioner* 208:254-258, 1972.

A. Nordenberg, G. Delisle, and T. Izukawa, "Cardiac Arrhythmia in a Child Due to Chloral Hydrate Ingestion." *Pediatrics* 47:134-135, 1971.

A. G. Robinson, and J. N. Loeb, "Ethanol Ingestion: Commonest Cause of Elevated Plasma Osmolality?" *N. Engl. J. Med.* 284:1253-1255, 1971.

CHAPTER 9

ANTIPSYCHOTIC TRANQUILIZERS AND ANTIDEPRESSANTS

Antipsychotic tranquilizers and antidepressants have revolutionized the treatment of mental illness, but they have also introduced new toxins for accidental ingestion by children and for adults who want to commit suicide. Cyclic antidepressants alone account for 37 percent of all poison-related admissions to intensive care units and for as much as 17 percent of all drug overdose deaths in the United States. The phenothiazine tranquilizers, first used in Europe in the late 1940s, have also gained enormous popularity. These drugs were first synthesized in the late 1800s during the development of aniline dyes in the textile industry. In the search for new antihistamines, early phenothiazine prototypes such as promethazine were found to have antihistaminic properties, and in fact both the phenothiazines and the tricyclic antidepressants are structurally similar to antihistamines. Although a discussion of antidepressants could include stimulants such as amphetamine and methylphenidate, these have been discussed in Chapter 7. The cyclic antidepressants are similar to the antipsychotic tranquilizers; thus both antipsychotic tranquilizers and cyclic antidepressants are discussed in this chapter (see Chap. 4 for laboratory determinations).

TRANQUILIZERS

In Europe antipsychotic tranquilizers are still called *neuroleptic drugs*. They can be divided into phenothiazine tranquilizers such as chlorpromazine (Thorazine) and nonphenothiazine tranquilizers such as haloperidol (Haldol) and hydroxyzine (Atarax). The tricyclic drug system of the phenothiazine is not essential to their effect.

The mechanism of action of the phenothiazines is not entirely understood, but they seem to increase dopamine turnover and to be cholinolytic in the central nervous system. The combined central effect is that of sedation that does not progress to anesthesia, as in the pure central nervous system depressants (see Chaps. 5 and 8). However, the phenothiazines ultimately produce seizures. They also have an autonomic parasympatholytic effect, but the expected pupillary dilatation and tachycardia may not always appear. In fact, bradycardia (slow conduction) and ectopic ventricular beat may occur. Pupillary constriction instead of mydriasis as well as postural hypotension due to an agonist effect on the beta-adrenergic (vasodilating) effect of endogenous epinephrine may also occur. Other effects are nonpuerperal lactation due to decreased production of hypothalamic prolactin inhibitory factor, pigmentary retinopathy, anterior lens cataract, and cholestatic jaundice. Table 9-1 shows the extrapyramidal effects these drugs tend to produce.

TABLE 9-1: EXTRAPYRAMIDAL EFFECTS

	Extrapyramidal Symptoms	Anticholinergic Effects
Phenothiazines: Aliphatic		
Chlorpromazine (Thorazine)	+	+ +
Promazine (Sparine)	+	+ +
Triflupromazine (Vesprin)	+	+ +
Phenothiazines: Piperidine		
Thioridazine (Mellaril)	±	+ +
Mesoridazine (Serentil)	±	+
Phenothiazines: Piperazine		
Acetophenazine (Tindal)	+ +	±
Perphenazine (Trilafon)	+ +	±
Prochlorperazine	+ +	±
Fluphenazine (Prolixin)	+ +	±
Trifluoperazine (Stelazine)	+ +	±
Thioxanthenes		
Chlorprothixene (Taractan)	±	+
Thiothixene (Navane)	+ +	±
Butyrophenone		
Haloperidol (Haldol)	+ +	±
Dihydroindolone		
Molindone (Moban)	+	+
Dibenzoxazepine		
Loxapine (Loxitane)	+ +	±

+ + = high; + = moderate; ± = low.

Poisoning

Acute poisoning. Acute poisoning with the phenothiazines leads to postural hypotension and peripheral autonomic parasympatholytic effects such as tachycardia, dryness of the mouth, and mydriasis with blurred vision. However, as previously stated, the pupils may also be constricted and bradycardia rather than tachycardia may ensue. A quinidinelike effect on the heart may be demonstrated on an electrocardiogram, with slow conduction and ventricular ectopic beat that may progress to ventricular arrhythmia and sudden death. Convulsions as well as parkinsonian equivalent signs such as opisthotonos and stiffness in the neck may also occur. These extrapyramidal signs of stiffness in the neck and other dystonia such as oculogyration and akathisia seem to be idiosyncratic rather than dose or allergy related.

Chronic poisoning. The prolonged use of the phenothiazines is fairly safe and has revolutionized psychiatric treatment. However, the phenothiazines may produce obstructive liver damage with inflammatory changes in the liver but without primary hepatic cell damage. They may also produce maculopapular eruptions, leukopenia or agranulocytosis, anterior lens capsule cataract, pigmentary retinopathy, nonpuerperal lactation, hyperpigmentation of the skin, and extrapyramidal signs and symptoms (see Table 9-1), which may occur in tardive dyskinesia even years after a therapeutic dose of phenothiazine has been discontinued.

Treatment

The general principles of treatment of acute overdose of a phenothiazine are described in Chapter 2. Methods to prevent continued absorption are particularly important, since these drugs slow gastric emptying and intestinal motility.

Specifically, that the hypotension that may occur with phenothiazine by placing the patient in shock position, that is, with the feet elevated, and by maintaining an adequate circulating volume. Some situations require plasma or plasma expanders. Sympathomimetic amines, with the exception of drugs without beta-adrenergic effect such as norepinephrine, are not beneficial in elevating the blood pressure. Furthermore, any sympathomimetic amine may increase the possibility of ventricular arrhythmia in these patients. Thus, use sympathomimetic amines, if required, with caution.

Diphenhydramine and other antiparkinson drugs will reverse promptly acute extrapyramidal signs and symptoms. Seizures require anticonvulsant therapy and conventional anticonvulsant drugs, such as diazepam and phenobarbital. Stop the drug at the first signs of jaundice, ocular changes, and bone marrow depression.

CYCLIC ANTIDEPRESSANTS

One of the most serious kinds of poisoning in the United States today, in both children and adults, arises from the wide usage and increasing accessibility of antidepressant drugs. These are not only the tricyclic antidepressants specifically used as antidepressants, but also drugs such as imipramine (Tofranil), which is widely used in pediatrics to treat patients with enuresis. Acute poisoning with these drugs is common, and the incidence is increasing.

The first antidepressant drugs developed were tricyclic in chemical structure, the newer derivatives may be bicyclic, tetracyclic (e.g., maprotiline) or of a miscellaneous structure that no longer resembles the original tricyclic nucleus. Members of the cyclic antidepressant group include imipramine, first used in Europe in 1958, desipramine, amitriptyline (Elavil), nortriptyline (Aventyl), doxepin (Sinequan), and maprotiline (Ludiomil). Table 9-2 lists the relation of structure to generic name.

TABLE 9-2: INTERRELATIONSHIP BETWEEN STRUCTURE AND ANTIDEPRESSANT

ANTIDEPRESSANT	STRUCTURAL CLASSIFICATION
Amitriptyline (Elavil)	Tricyclic
Amoxapine (Asendin)	Tricyclic
Desipramine (Norpramin)	Tricyclic
Doxepin (Sinequan)	Tricyclic
Imipramine (Tofranil)	Tricyclic
Loxapine (Loxitane)	Tricyclic
Maprotiline (Ludiomil)	Tetracyclic
Nortriptyline (Aventyl)	Tricyclic
Protriptyline (Vivactil)	Tricyclic
Trazodone (Desyrel)	Miscellaneous
Trimipramine (Surmontil)	Tricyclic

Cyclic antidepressant compounds are absorbed rapidly and quickly become firmly tissue bound, so that the blood level is always relatively low. Efficient detoxification occurs in the liver, and very little active drug appears in the urine. In therapeutic doses elimination occurs rapidly; scarcely any of the parent drug remains in the tissues 24 hours after ingestion.

Cyclic antidepressants are toxic in even small amounts, but their precise mechanism of action is incompletely known. They act by blocking acetylcholine-mediated transmitters in the central nervous system and by a powerful anticholinergic effect in the peripheral tissues. The peripheral toxic effects therefore resemble those of atropinism with resultant tachycardia, which if severe may cause hypotension. More severe arrhythmias and cardiac conduction disorders, which may occur in serious cyclic overdosage, cannot be attributed to the anticholinergic action and may result from a direct toxic effect on the myocardium or by interference with norepinephrine release from cardiac nerve endings.

The cyclic antidepressants stimulate the central nervous system, which can lead to convulsion as well as parasympatholytic effects such as dryness of the mouth and mydriasis. They also produce severe cardiac arrhythmias, worse than those caused by most parasympatholytic agents, including the phenothiazines. The minimum lethal dose is approximately 30 mg/kg. These drugs are mostly metabolized in the liver. The first 24 hours are crucial in survival.

Poisoning

Acute poisoning. Acute poisoning with cyclic antidepressants, as previously mentioned, produces clinical manifestations of parasympathetic block including mydriasis and dryness of the mouth. Patients may also have severe central nervous system stimulation associated with convulsions, hallucinations, respiratory depression, and fall in blood pressure. However, the most significant problem is the seriousness of the cardiac arrhythmias.

These cardiac arrhythmias include atrial and nodal tachycardia as well as atrioventricular block, bundle branch block, and other intraventricular conduction disorders. The electrocardiogram may show widening of the QRS deflection, depressed ST deflection, abnormal T wave, and evidence of supraventricular tachycardia and even of ventricular tachycardia. The final outcome can be hypotension and cardiac arrest.

These features appear 1 to 6 hours after overdose and seldom last longer than 18 to 24 hours, but sudden death has been reported up to 6 days after ingestion of the cyclic drug. Ingestion of more than 10 mg/kg of most of the cyclic antidepressant drugs has resulted in serious toxicity, with doses greater than 35 mg/kg associated with death. In children, refer any ingestion for observation for at least 6 hours in an emergency facility. If a patient remains asymptomatic for this period, it is unlikely that ingestion occurred. If symptoms develop, the patient should be admitted and monitored for a minimum of 48 hours.

Chronic poisoning. Chronic overuse of cyclic antidepressants also leads to clinical manifestations of atropinism such as dryness of the mouth, blurred vision due to mydriasis, and urinary retention. These patients may also show lethargy, convulsions, agitation with exacerbation of schizophrenic symptoms, and cardiac arrhythmias. The various formulations of antidepressant drugs produce differing degrees of central nervous system and cardiac involvement depending on their structural classification. Table 9-2 gives the different structural classifications for the more popular antidepressants.

Treatment

General principles have been outlined in Chapter 2. Methods to prevent continued absorption are particularly important, since these drugs slow gastric emptying and intestinal motility. Perform emesis if it can be done quickly, before symptoms of central nervous system depression develop. Forced diuresis, peritoneal dialysis, and hemodialysis, as in phenothiazine treatment, are of little or no value because these drugs are tissue and protein bound. Hemoperfusion has not been used enough to determine its effectiveness. The treatment of hypotension described for phenothiazine also applies to cyclic antidepressants, since they also produce hypotension by increasing the beta-adrenergic effect of endogenous epinephrine. Furthermore, use sympathomimetic amines, when required, with even more caution than in phenothiazine overdose because the possibility of ventricular arrhythmias is even greater.

Patients with ventricular arrhythmias that do not respond to alkalinization and phenytoin may respond to lidocaine, propranolol, or physostigmine. Seizures normally respond well to conventional anticonvulsants (e.g., diazepam or phenytoin). If seizures are refractory, use physostigmine. If physostigmine is used, keep atropine sulfate available to counteract side effects that may occur. Parasympathomimetic drugs such as physostigmine may be valuable in counteracting the parasympatholytic effect of cyclic antidepressants at certain times, but reserve physostigmine for use when conventional drugs fail. Some parasympathomimetic drugs are quaternary amines and do not cross the blood-brain barrier, but physostigmine is a tertiary amine and thus crosses the blood-brain barrier, countering the central stimulant effect of the cyclic antidepressants.

References — Chapter 9

M. D. Allen, D. J. Greenblatt, and B. O. Noel, "Overdosage with Antipsychotic Agents." *Psychiatry* 137:234-239, 1980.

J. M. Arena, "Two Current Poisonings: Tricyclic Drugs and Methadone." *Pediatrics* 51:919, 1973.

M. T. Boehnert, and F. H. Lovejoy, "Value of the ORS Duration Versus the Serum Drug Level in Predicting Seizures and Ventricular Arrhythmias after an Acute Overdose of Tricyclic Antidepressants." *N. Engl. J. of Med.* 313:474-479, 1985.

O. Chadovam, and S. Chatharpt, "Treatment of Chlorpromazine Poisoning with Naloxone." *J. Pediatr.* 106:515-516, 1985.

H. N. Donnewald, "L'intoxication algue par les phenothiazines chez l'adulte, a propos de 112 cas." *Eur. J. Toxicol.* 3:167-178, 1970.

E. L. Dubois, E. Tallman, and R. A. Wonka, "Chlorpromazine-Induced Systemic Lupus Erythematosus." *J.A.M.A.* 221:595-596, 1972.

B. Duffy, "Acute Phenothiazine Intoxication in Children." *Med. J. Aust.* 1:676-678, 1971.

J. P. Fréjaville, et al., "Intoxications aigue par les amines phenothiziniques, a propos de 152 cas." *Eur. J. Toxicol.* 3:179-187, 1970.

J. W. Jefferson, and J. H. Greist, "Some Hazards of Lithium Use." *Am. J. Psychiatry* 138:93-97, 1981.

H. Matthew, "Acute Poisoning with Antidepressant Drugs: Treatment of Common Acute Poisoning," 3rd ed. (London: Longman, 1975), pp. 81-83.

M. Tsuang, et al., "Haloperidol Versus Thiordazine for Hospitalized Psychogeriatric Patients: Double-Blind Study." *J. Am. Geriatr. Soc.* 19:593-600, 1971.

CHAPTER **10** *XANTHINE DERIVATIVES*

Theophylline, caffeine, and theobromine are three widely consumed alkaloids that occur in plants. Tea is one beverage-producing plant that contains all three chemicals. These three drugs share important pharmacologic actions: stimulation of the central nervous system, action on the kidney to produce diuresis, stimulation of heart muscle, and relaxation of smooth muscle, particularly bronchial muscle. Only caffeine and theophylline have therapeutic and toxicologic importance and will be discussed here.

CAFFEINE

The most important source of caffeine is the fruit of the plant Coffea arabica and related species. The beverage made from the dried and processed fruit or bean has been used since ancient times as a mood elevator and stimulant. In modern times it has been incorporated into numerous stimulant and analgesic formulations. Caffeine is believed to enhance analgesia when used in combination with pain-relieving drugs. Chemically it is 1,3,7 trimethylxanthine.

Poisoning

Acute poisoning. In adults, a single large dose of 1 g of caffeine will produce confusion, tremors, tachycardia, fever, vomiting, and diarrhea. Lethal dose in an adult is estimated to be about 10 g. Large doses of caffeine can produce insomnia, restlessness, tinnitus, and convulsions. Headaches, nausea, vomiting, miosis, alternating states of consciousness, low-grade fever, photophobia, and delirium have also been reported following large doses. Cardiovascular effects include sinus tachycardia, bigeminy, paroxysmal atrial tachycardia, and premature ventricular contractions. Death from cardiovascular collapse has occurred following massive doses. Respiratory arrest can occur with massive doses. Low to moderate doses will produce urination with associated fluid loss. With very severe caffeine intoxication, gastrointestinal hemorrhages, possibly accompanied by seizures, can develop. Hyperglycemia, hypokalemia, ketonuria, metabolic acidosis, and markedly elevated norepinephrine and epinephrine plasma levels have been reported. Death following caffeine overdose is rare but has occurred. Caffeine's popularity in "kiddy dope" and "look-alike" preparations has contributed to an increase in reportings of toxic effects from this drug.

Chronic poisoning. Excessive consumption of coffee and stimulants containing caffeine causes gastric irritation, nausea, and vomiting. Low to moderate doses will produce urination. Sudden withdrawal from beverages containing caffeine can result in a headache that is relieved by administration of caffeine.

Treatment

Initiate standard methods to prevent absorption (see Chap. 2). Treat seizures with intravenous diazepam, 0.1 to 0.3 mg/kg in a child and up to 10 mg in an adult. If the patient remains unresponsive, administer phenytoin, 15 mg/kg intravenously no faster than 0.5 mg/kg/min while monitoring the electrocardiogram. Monitor urinary output carefully and replace fluid as needed. Carotid sinus massage is helpful in reverting paroxysmal atrial tachycardia. Depending on type and severity, treat arrhythmias with the appropriate agent (e.g., lidocaine, phenytoin). Treat gastrointestinal irritation with a demulcent such as aluminum hydroxide gel.

THEOPHYLLINE

Theophylline, 1,3 dimethylxanthine, is widely used in children and adults to stimulate and promote breathing in asthma. The drug is frequently involved in iatrogenic overdoses.

Poisoning

Acute poisoning. Insomnia, nervousness, and irritability are common following initial administration of the drug even in therapeutic amounts. Tolerance to these adverse effects usually develops with continued usage. Sustained-release preparations are typically used for persons who must maintain steady-state blood levels of theophylline. Overdosage with sustained-release preparations of theophylline results in severe and prolonged central nervous system and cardiovascular toxicity associated with sustained toxic serum levels. Overdosage with sustained-action preparations is more severe than with conventional preparations and is probably due to large doses being absorbed over extended periods. Nausea, vomiting, headaches, abdominal cramps, and diarrhea occur when the serum concentration of theophylline rises above 20 micrograms/ml. Severe toxicity includes severe restlessness, agitation, seizures, cardiac arrhythmias including atrial fibrillation and ventricular tachycardia, and cardiac arrest.

Chronic poisoning. All the manifestations of acute poisoning occur if the blood level exceeds therapeutic. Theophylline-induced diuresis may lead to hypokalemia, especially if accompanied by vomiting. Dehydration may also occur.

Treatment

Use all standard procedures for preventing absorption. Additionally, gastric dialysis, and giving repeated doses of activated charcoal, may be particularly useful for patients who have overdosed on time-release formulations of theophylline. Treat seizures, which may be refractory to standard anticonvulsant therapy and may not abate until theophylline levels decline. Administer diazepam intravenously. If seizures are uncontrolled, give undiluted phenytoin in an intravenous push or dilute 50 mg/ml in 50 to 100 ml of normal saline. Administer 15 to 18 mg/kg intravenously no faster than 0.5 mg/kg/min or 50 mg/min while monitoring the electrocardiogram. Stop or slow the infusion rate if hypotension or arrhythmias occur. If seizures are still refractory, administer phenobarbital or pentobarbital. Repeat as needed unless hypotension occurs. If seizures are still refractory, or if 20 to 60 minutes have gone by, consider general anesthesia with halothane or thiopental or paralysis with curare or pancuronium bromide, requiring intubation and mechanical ventilation. Obtain a serum theophylline level. Monitor patients with a serum level above 20 micrograms/ml and signs of toxicity until the level reaches the therapeutic range. If the patient is hypotensive, administer intravenous fluids and place in the Trendelenburg position. Try to avoid pressor agents if possible. If the patient is unresponsive to these measures, administer dopamine or levarterenol. Administer 2 to 5 micrograms/kg/min of dopamine, progressing as needed to as high as 50 micrograms/kg/min. If ventricular arrhythmias occur, decrease the rate of administration.

For levarterenol begin at 0.1 to 0.2 micrograms/kg/min and increase as needed. Monitor cardiac function closely. For ventricular tachycardia, use lidocaine intravenously followed by an intravenous drip.

      For supraventricular tachycardia institute one of the following: verapamil, digitalization, or propranolol in a *nonasthmatic* patient. Do not use propranolol in an asthmatic patient because it may potentiate the asthma. Use propranolol as follows: Adult, 1 mg intravenously every 2 to 5 minutes until a response is seen or a maximum of 10 mg has been given; child, 0.01 to 0.1 mg/kg/dose intravenously every 2 to 5 minutes until a response is seen or a maximum of 1 mg has been given. If propranolol is the only treatment that can be used, have Isuprel ready to infuse to counteract the propranolol. Consider metoprolol or atenolol in an asthmatic patient but not in a child. Consider administering procainamide or quinidine for supraventricular tachycardia or arrhythmias. Follow the same regimen for arrhythmias as for tachycardia. Provide full support and hydration while the drug is being metabolized. Since only small amounts of theophylline are excreted by renal mechanisms, forced diuresis is ineffective in enhancing elimination of theophylline. Theophylline is metabolized rapidly enough so that dialysis normally is not warranted. However, at blood theophylline levels above 60 micrograms/ ml, activated charcoal hemoperfusion has been recommended if toxic signs and symptoms are severe. Hemodialysis also has been reported to increase the elimination of theophylline, with a clearance of 24 mg/kg/hr being achieved. Exchange transfusion may be useful in severely intoxicated neonates and infants in whom hemoperfusion cannot be performed.

References — Chapter 10

P. Baltassat, et al., "Theophylline: Acute Poisoning in a Child. Evidence for Biotransformation of Theophylline into Caffeine." *Vet. Hum. Toxicol.* 21(Suppl):211, 1979.

W. S. Brukle, and C. J. Gwizdala, "Evaluation of 'Toxic' Serum Theophylline Concentrations." *Am. J. Hosp. Pharm.* 38:1164, 1981.

J. M. C. Connell, et al., "Self-Poisoning with Sustained-Release Aminophylline: Secondary Rise in Serum Theophylline Concentration after Charcoal Haemoperfusion." *Br. Med. J.* 284:943, 1982.

P. Gal, et al., "Theophylline-Induced Seizures in Accidentally Overdosed Neonates." *Pediatrics* 65:547, 1980.

M. Helliwell, and D. Berry, "Theophylline Poisoning in Adults." *Br. Med. J.* 2:1114, 1979.

L. Hendeles, and M. Weinberger, "Poisoning Patients with Intravenous Theophylline." *Am. J. Hosp. Pharmacol.* 37:49, 1980.

D. B. Jeffreys, et al., "Haemoperfusion for Theophylline Overdose." *Br. Med. J.* 280:1167, 1980.

J. N. Miceli, A. Bidani, and R. Aronow, "Peritoneal Dialysis of Theophylline." *Clin. Toxicol.* 14:539, 1979.

CHAPTER 11 PARASYMPATHOLYTICS AND ANTIHISTAMINES

Parasympatholytic (or anticholinergic) compounds such as atropine mainly block the parasympathomimetic or muscarinic effects of acetylcholine not only distal to the parasympathetic nerve endings but also at the motor end plates and in the brain and thus prevent the action of acetylcholine on smooth and skeletal muscle, glands, heart, and brain. Following the principle of the atropine-acetylcholine antagonism, drugs were developed to counteract the action of histamine by competitive antagonism. Antihistamine drugs have mainly peripheral histamine-blocking action but also have some central nervous system effects.

PARASYMPATHOLYTIC AGENTS

The therapeutic usefulness of the parasympatholytic drugs, as well as the ease with which synthetic analogs of the natural occurring alkaloid can be produced, has resulted in a large number of these compounds in home medicine chests.

The natural occurring alkaloids are atropine, which comes from the shrub *Atropa belladonna*; and scopolamine and related alkaloids, which come from henbane, *Hyoscyamus niger*, and from jimson weed, *Datura stramonium*.

All the natural occurring alkaloids are tertiary amines. The synthetic analogs are either tertiary amines such as benztropine (Cogentin) or quaternary ammonium compounds such as propantheline (Pro-Banthine). The tertiary compounds cross the blood-brain barrier; the quaternary compounds do not and therefore have no central nervous system effect.

Parasympatholytics are competitive antagonists of acetylcholine at the receptor site and therefore induce tachycardia, relax all nonvascular smooth muscle, and decrease secretory activities of all exocrine glands such as sweat glands. Furthermore, those compounds that cross the blood-brain barrier (tertiary amines) produce a peculiar central nervous system sedation associated with amnesia, excitement, delirium, and even convulsions.

Poisoning

Acute poisoning. Acute intoxication with parasympatholytic drugs and plants containing these compounds (Table 11-1) causes dryness of the mouth, tachycardia, hot, dry, red skin, fever, urinary retention, mydriasis and blurred vision, muscle stiffness, delirium, and convulsions. Respiratory depression may occur with scopolamine.

TABLE 11-1: PARASYMPATHOLYTICS AND ANTIHISTAMINES

THERAPEUTIC OR PHARMACOLOGIC CLASS	DRUG EXAMPLE
Antihistamines	Chlorpheniramine (Chlor-Trimeton) diphenhydramine (Benadryl) promethazine (Phenergan)
Antispasmodics	Methantheline (Banthine) propantheline (Probanthine)
Antipsychotic tranquilizers	Phenothiazines (e.g., Mellaril) butyrophenones (e.g., Haldol)
Antiparkinson agents	Benztropine mesylate (Cogentin)
Ophthalmic preparations	Atropine (various brands)
Cyclic antidepressants	Amitriptyline HCL (Elavil) desipramine HCL (Norpramin) Doxepin HCL (Sinequan) Imipramine HCL (Tofranil)
Plants	Deadly nightshade (*Atropa belladonna*) Jimsonweed (*Datura stromonium*) Jerusalem cherry (*Solanum pseudocapsicum*)

Chronic poisoning. Repeated exposure to these compounds, as in acute intoxication, may cause dryness of the mouth, hot, dry, red skin, fever, urinary retention, mydriasis and blurred vision, muscle stiffness, and even delirium.

Treatment

Emergency measures after overexposure to these drugs or to plants containing these compounds are described in Chapter 2. The specific pharmacologic antagonists for these compounds are the parasympathomimetic drugs such as physostigmine (see Chaps. 2 and 9). However, exercise caution when using these agents.

Symptomatic supportive care is always important (see Chap. 2) and may be preferable to the use of physostigmine for minimal to moderate exposure. For example, institute sponge bathing to reduce fever, anticonvulsant therapy for convulsions, and good hydration with bladder catheterization if the patient is unable to void. Major tranquilizers such as the phenothiazines do not help the delirium the parasympatholytic drugs cause.

ANTIHISTAMINES

The antihistamines were developed, with the atropine acetylcholine model in mind, to counteract the effect of histamine. The antihistamines, as well as the parasympatholytic and antipsychotic drugs, have similar basic chemical configurations. The antihistamines, however, are further classified into five subgroups: ethanolamines, ethylenediamines, phenothiazines, alkylamines, and piperidines. A new subgroup, "miscellaneous," accommodates the recently introduced antihistamine terfenadine (Seldane). In any case, the primary effect of counteracting histamine is shared by all antihistamines. In addition, most antihistamines share common side effects. The major side effect of antihistamines is a peculiar central nervous system depression or sedation that, like that produced by the parasympatholytic drugs, is associated with signs of stimulation including delirium and convulsions. Some of the antihistamines such as diphenhydramine, usually produce more marked central nervous system depression. Just as the parasympatholytics are not innocuous drugs, neither are the antihistamines. This, of course, is contrary to popular belief if one considers the enormous indiscriminate use of these drugs, particularly in children under 5 years of age. Antihistamines are listed in Table 11-2.

TABLE 11-2: ANTIHISTAMINES

GENERIC NAME	BRAND NAME	CHEMICAL CLASS	DURATION (HRS)
Diphenhydramine	Benadryl	Ethanolamine	4-6
Tripelennamine	Pyribenzamine	Ethylenediamine	4-6
Chlorpheniramine	Chlor-Trimeton	Alkylamine	4-6
Brompheniramine	Dimetane	Alkylamine	4-6
Cyproheptadine	Periactin	Piperidine	4-6
Promethazine	Phenergan	Phenothiazine	4-6
Clemastine	Tavist	Ethanolamine	4-6
Terfenadine	Seldane	Miscellaneous	10-12

Poisoning.

Acute poisoning. Acute intoxication with antihistamines produces atropinelike effects: tachycardia, dryness of the mouth, urinary retention, and drowsiness and mydriasis. Hallucination, stupor, tremors, and even convulsions may also occur. These effects may begin to occur with doses over 10 mg/kg for the ethanolamine-type antihistamines. It is difficult to predict toxicity based on milligram per kilogram ingested amounts because potency varies based on the type of antihistamine. The most common toxic effects reported in one poison center study of calls on antihistamine exposure in children under 5 years of age are listed here in order of frequency: drowsiness, vomiting, lethargy, mydriasis, hyperactivity, irritability, flushing, ataxia, nausea, diarrhea, tachycardia, and slurred speech.

Chronic poisoning. The chronic use of antihistamines leads to toxic effects similar to those seen in acute intoxication. Furthermore, some antihistamines such as tripelennamine have been reported to cause bone marrow depression.

Treatment

The principles of emergency care are described in Chapter 2. There are no definitive specific antidotes. General supportive measures are of course essential. Major tranquilizers, as in treatment of poisoning from the parasympatholytic drugs, are not useful in treating the hallucinations caused by antihistamines. The seizures must be treated with anticonvulsants such as phenobarbital and diazepam. If coma and respiratory depression occur, treat them with mechanical assistance rather than with stimulant drugs, which may precipitate convulsions.

References — Chapter 11

M. Bloomquist, et al., "Lethal Orphenadrine Intoxications." *Z. Rechtsmedizin* 68:111-114, 1971.

R. E. Bluhm, and W. C. Koller, "Anticholinergic Abuse." *Drug Ther.* 11:150-155, 1981.

A. Fatteh, and J. B. Dudley, "Fatal Poisoning Involving Methapyrilene." *J.A.M.A.* 219:756-757, 1972.

R. G. Hooper, C. S. Conner, and B. H. Rumack, "Acute Poisonings from Over-the-Counter Sleep Preparations," *J. Am. Coll. Emergency Phys.* 8:98-100, 1979.

J. Kalivas, "Cyproheptadine-Induced Photosensitivity." *J.A.M.A.* 216:526, 1971.

K. M. Leighton, "Paranoid Psychosis After Abuse of Actifed." *Br. Med. J.* 284:789-791, 1982.

R. Malcolm, and W. C. Miller, "Dimenhydrinate (Dramamine) Abuse: Hallucinogenic Experiences with a Proprietary Antihistamine." *Am. J. Psychiatr.* 128:1012-1013, 1972.

Y. Soleymanikashi, and M. S. Weiss, "Antihistaminic Reactions: A Review and Presentation of 2 Unusual Examples." *Ann. Allergy* 28:486-490, 1970.

D. L. Uden, et al., "Antihistamines: A Study of Pediatric Usage and Incidence of Toxicity." *Vet. Hum. Toxicol.* 26:469-472, 1984.

S. West, et al., "A Review of Antihistamines and the Common Cold." *Pediatrics* 56:100-107, 1975.

CHAPTER 12 *CARDIOVASCULAR DRUGS*

It is difficult to consolidate all cardiovascular drugs into one chapter because these agents differ extensively in their pharmacology and toxicology. Since cardiovascular diseases lead the list of illnesses in the United States, the 1980s have seen a proliferation of cardioactive agents available to the clinician in treating heart disease. As a result, these drugs are ubiquitous in home medicine chests.

CARDIAC GLYCOSIDES

Cardiac glycosides are used therapeutically in heart failure because of their positive chronotropic and inotropic effects on the heart. Because of these powerful effects on the myocardium, they are unrivaled for their value in the treatment of heart failure.

Poisoning

Acute poisoning. Ingestion of 2 mg or more of digoxin (Lanoxin) has been reported to cause toxicity in adults. It is not possible from the literature to determine the minimum toxic or lethal dose in humans. However, less than 2 mg in patients receiving chronic digoxin therapy may result in toxicity.

Nausea and vomiting are symptoms of acute and chronic toxicity. Visual disturbances including photophobia, amblyopia, aberrations of color vision, and scotoma may occur. Lethargy, drowsiness, weakness, paresthesias, and headache may occur. Profound hyperkalemia, which may be life threatening, may result from acute poisoning. This is unlike chronic poisoning, which is generally associated with hypokalemia due to concurrent diuretic administration where potassium leaks out of the cell over a long period. Cardiac dysrhythmias of every known type have been associated with digitalis intoxication.

Chronic poisoning. Chronic toxicity from cardiac glycosides is frequent in adults and may be severe or even fatal. Approximately 25 percent of hospitalized patients taking cardiac glycosides show some signs of toxicity. The most frequent cause of toxicity with cardiac glycosides is the concurrent administration of diuretics that cause potassium depletion. All the cardiac effects mentioned under acute poisoning can occur from chronic malcompliance with dosage regimens, since patients must be maintained at steady-state blood levels.

Treatment

Prevent absorption as discussed in Chapter 2. Monitor the electrocardiogram continuously for abnormal cardiac rates and rhythms. Consider inserting a transvenous pacemaker in those patients with severe bradycardia or slow ventricular rate due to second degree atrioventricular block who fail to respond to atropine or phenytoin drug therapy.

Hyperkalemia following acute overdose may be life threatening. Management includes intravenous administration of sodium bicarbonate, glucose, and insulin. Kayexalate also lowers serum potassium levels. Atropine is useful in managing bradycardia, varying degrees of heart block, and other cardiac irregularities. Low-dose phenytoin may improve atrioventricular conduction. Larger doses are needed to manage ventricular dysrhythmias. Lidocaine is useful in managing ventricular tachyarrhythmias, premature ventricular contractions, and bigeminy. Hemodialysis is ineffective in removing cardiac glycosides but may help to restore potassium levels to normal.

Antigen binding fragments (FAB) distributed under the brand name Digibind, manufactured by Burroughs Wellcome Company, have shown promise in children and adults in reversing digoxin and digitoxin overdose. Most childhood ingestions would not warrant the use of FAB fragments. These antibodies are indicated for life-threatening manifestations of digoxin and digitoxin overdose. Manifestations of life-threatening toxicity include:

1. *Severe* ventricular dysrhythmias, including ventricular tachycardia or ventricular fibrillation which do not respond to first line treatment.

2. Progressive bradydysrhythmias, including *severe* sinus bradycardia (not just mild prolongation of P-R, or ST-T changes); or, 2° or 3° degree heart block not responsive to atropine.

3. Ingestions of 10 mg of digoxin in previously healthy adults or 4 mg in children or ingestions resulting in steady-state serum concentrations >10 ng/ml may result in cardiac arrest. These patients may be candidates for FAB fragment treatment.

4. Elevated serum potassium as a result of digitalis toxicity indicates imminent cardiac arrest. Patients with serum potassium levels >5-6.0 mEq/1 in the setting of digitalis toxicity are candidates for FAB fragment treatment.

For dosing, administration, precautions, and additional information, use the product package insert from the manufacturer or contact a regional poison center for assistance. Digibind is available at strategically located hospitals throughout the United States. For information on its availability in any area the regional poison center should be contacted. The poison center will also have available toll-free numbers for manufacturer assistance.

VASODILATOR ANTIHYPERTENSIVE DRUGS

By convention, vasodilators are those drugs that act to dilate blood vessels by direct action on the smooth muscle of the vascular system. Hydralazine (Apresoline), diazoxide (Hyperstat IV), minoxidil (Loniten), the thiazides (Diuril, Hydrodiuril), nitroprusside (Nipride), and prazosin (Minipress) are all members of this class.

Poisoning

Acute poisoning. Small to moderate acute overdoses of hydralazine, minoxidil, prazosin, and the thiazides have not been reported to cause significant toxicity. Hydralazine and diazoxide both cause reflex activation of the sympathetic nervous system so that tachycardia may occur. However, more frequently drowsiness and even profound lack of reflexes without hypotension have been reported with large overdoses. Children have tolerated as much as 50 mg of prazosin in a single dose with only minimal effects. Neurologically, headache and dizziness may occur. With prazosin therapy, fainting may occur with a change in dosage or an excessive initial dose. Gastrointestinal effects include nausea and vomiting.

Chronic poisoning. Chronic effects of these agents are more related to their side effects than to toxicity from long-term use. The cardiovascular system is most affected. Excessive hypotension and reflex sympathetic stimulation can occur. Hydralazine has become more widely used since beta blockers were introduced; concomitant use of these drugs blocks sympathetic reflex activity, making beta blockers effective in smaller doses for longer periods with fewer side effects.

Treatment

Institute the methods to prevent absorption discussed in Chapter 2. If the patient is hypotensive, administer intravenous fluids and place the patient in the Trendelenburg position. If the patient is unresponsive to these measures, administer dopamine or levarterenol. In patients displaying severe symptoms, monitor central venous or pulmonary wedge pressure. Closely follow renal function. Maintain an adequate urine output but do not force diuresis. Reverse diazoxide-induced hyperglycemia with either insulin or oral hypoglycemic agents. Treat peripheral neuropathies, most commonly associated with long-term therapeutic doses of hydralazine, with pyridoxine. Priapism requires *immediate* consultation with a urologic surgeon.

BETA-ADRENERGIC BLOCKING AGENTS

Propranolol (Inderal) is the prototypical and still most important beta-adrenergic blocking agent. Other drugs in this group are nadolol (Corgard), pindolol (Visken), and timolol (Blocadren). These are nonselective beta blockers that block receptors in bronchial smooth muscle and skeletal muscle, thereby interfering with bronchodilatation produced by epinephrine and other sympathomimetic amines. The more selective blockers include metoprolol (Lopressor), atenolol (Tenormin) and acebutolol (Sectral). These drugs, whose selectivity is dose related, are less likely to affect bronchodilatation. All the drugs have a similar effect but differ considerably in bioavailability and pharmacokinetics. The beta blockers are indicated in the treatment of cardiac arrhythmias, hypertrophic subaortic stenosis, pheochromocytoma, hypertension, migraine, and angina pectoris.

Poisoning

Acute poisoning. Poisoning from acute overdose of these agents is related to cardiac blockade. Acute overdose can result in bradycardia, bronchospasm, hypotension, and complete heart block.

Chronic poisoning. Chronic administration of these drugs can cause numerous adverse reactions. Many central nervous system and psychiatric effects have been reported, ranging from dizziness, fatigue, and vertigo to acute, profound mental changes; these are reversible with reduced dosage or discontinuance of the drug. Hyperglycemia and hypoglycemia have been reported. Numerous hematologic, endocrine, gastrointestinal, dermatologic, ophthalmologic, and respiratory effects have occurred with long-term administration.

Treatment

Begin methods to prevent absorption as discussed in Chapter 2 as soon as possible following ingestion. Monitor electrocardiographic and vital signs carefully for bradycardia and conduction defects. Bradycardia, conduction defects, and hypotension should respond to intravenous glucagon, atropine, isoproterenol, or transvenous pacing.

Glucagon may produce a positive chronotropic and inotropic cardiac effect, which occurs despite beta blockage. Dilute glucagon for this use with 5 percent dextrose in water instead of the diluent provided. Use atropine to reduce vagal stimulation and subsequently increase heart rate. Isoproterenol is a beta agonist that will competitively antagonize the effect of the beta blocker, but hypotension may be aggravated by isoproterenol, necessitating careful monitoring of blood pressure and titration of dose. Insert a transvenous pacemaker if heart block or severe bradycardia cannot be easily controlled with drugs. Manage hypoglycemia with intravenous glucose, glucagon, or both. Bronchoconstriction may require treatment with isoproterenol inhalation, which may require larger than usual doses, or aminophylline. Hemodialysis apparently is not useful because these drugs are greater than 95 percent protein bound, although nadolol and atenolol have been reported to be removed by hemodialysis.

CALCIUM CHANNEL BLOCKERS

Verapamil (Calan, Isoptin), nifedipine (Procardia), and diltiazem (Cardizem) are drugs that inhibit the movement of calcium ions across the cell membrane. The resulting pharmacologic effect on the cardiovascular system is to depress mechanical contraction of both myocardial and smooth muscle and depress electrical impulse formation and conduction velocity. These agents are indicated in various types of angina pectoris and are described in Table 12-1.

TABLE 12-1: CALCIUM CHANNEL BLOCKING AGENTS

GENERIC NAME	BRAND NAME	ONSET (MINS)	PEAK LEVEL (HRS)
Nifedipine	Procardia	20	0.5
Verapamil	Isoptin	30	1-2.2
Diltiazem	Cardizem	30	2-3

Poisoning

Acute poisoning. Small acute doses of the calcium channel blockers, the kind that typically occur in childhood ingestions, seem to be well tolerated. Large overdoses can cause excessive peripheral vasodilatation with subsequent prolonged hypotension. Asystole and heart block can occur with verapamil. There is limited information with acute overdosage of these agents, but single doses of diltiazem several times the total daily dose have been well tolerated in adults.

Chronic poisoning. Adverse reactions from these drugs are related to their unique effects on the cardiovascular system, and most are expected consequences of the vasodilator effects.

Treatment

Prevent absorption as discussed in Chapter 2. Monitor vital signs frequently. Initially treat hypotension and bradycardia with positioning. Administer calcium gluconate as a 10 percent solution if necessary, carefully monitoring the electrocardiogram and serum calcium level. Dopamine or norepinephrine may be used to treat hypotension. Heart block may respond to intravenous calcium, glucagon, or isoproterenol. Treat seizures with diazepam, phenytoin, or phenobarbital.

CENTRALLY ACTING ANTIHYPERTENSIVE AGENTS

The centrally acting antihypertensive agents include methyldopa (Aldomet), guanabenz (Wytensin) and clonidine (Catapres). The current thinking about central regulation of blood pressure stems from the observation that stimulating alpha-adrenergic receptors in the brain inhibits peripheral sympathetic activity, thus lowering blood pressure.

Poisoning

Acute poisoning. In acute overdose, methyldopa and guanabenz appear to be better tolerated than clonidine, although guanabenz has caused hypotension, somnolence, lethargy, irritability, miosis, and bradycardia following overdose in children under 5 years of age. Clonidine overdosage has produced bradycardia, central nervous system depression, respiratory depression, apnea, hypothermia, miosis, seizures, lethargy, agitation, irritability, diarrhea, and arrhythmias. Small overdoses of clonidine in children characteristically produce weakness, somnolence, diminished reflexes, and severe hypotension. The acute effects of clonidine in overdose and its chemistry are similar to the imidazoline sympathomimetics, such as tetrahydrozoline and naphazoline.

Chronic poisoning. Adverse effects from these drugs include central nervous system effects such as sedation, lightheadedness, and even psychic impairment. Cardiovascular effects are due to the pharmacologic effects of the drugs and include orthostatic hypotension, edema, and aggravation of angina. Gastrointestinal, hepatic, hematologic, and allergic reactions may occur.

Treatment

Patients with clonidine-induced apnea and coma have been reported to respond to naloxone. Administer an initial intravenous dose of 0.8 to 2 mg in either a child or an adult. Although it may exceed the manufacturer's recommendation, this dose level has been used successfully. Treat seizures with intravenous diazepam. If the patient is unresponsive, administer phenytoin while monitoring the electrocardiogram. Treat hypotension first by placing the patient in the Trendelenburg position and by volume expansion with isotonic fluids. If the patient is unresponsive to these measures, administer vasopressors, particularly dopamine. Bradycardia following clonidine overdosage may not be symptomatic and may not require treatment. Bradycardia and hypotension may respond to atropine alone. Although tolazoline (Priscoline) is reported to reverse bradycardia and hypotension secondary to clonidine, it is unpredictable and should be reserved for those patients who do not respond to fluids, dopamine, or atropine. Tolazoline is a complex drug and can cause marked hypertension, cardiac arrhythmias, and tachycardia. Give it at a dose of 10 mg intravenously, repeated every 5 to 10 minutes as needed up to a maximum of 40 mg. Exercise caution in treating hypertension; in life-threatening situations, use nitroprusside. Treat cardiac arrhythmias with standard antiarrhythmic drugs if necessary.

References — Chapter 12

A. Buiumsohn, et al., "Seizures and Intraventricular Conduction Defect in Propranolol Poisoning." *Ann. Intern. Med.* 91:860, 1979.

C. E. Drake, "Cardiac Drug Overdose." *Am. Fam. Physician* 25:181, 1982.

H. J. Gilfrich, et al., "Successful Treatment of Massive Digitoxin Overdose by Charcoal Hemoperfusion." *Vet. Hum. Toxicol.* 21(Suppl):18, 1979.

P. J. Halloran, and C. E. Phillips, "Propranolol Intoxication." *Arch. Intern. Med.* 141:810, 1981.

V. Hansteen, et al., "Acute, Massive Poisoning with Digitoxin: Report of Seven Cases and Discussion of Treatment." *Clin. Toxicol.* 18:679, 1981.

D. A. Henry, et al., "The Changing Pattern of Toxicity of Digitoxin." *Postgrad. Med. J.* 57:358, 1981.

K. Laake, et al., "Convulsions and Possible Spasm of the Lower Esophageal Sphincter in a Fatal Case of Propranolol Intoxication." *Acta Med. Scand.* 210:137, 1981.

R. E. Pieroni, and J. G. Fisher, "Use of Cholestyramine Resin in Digitoxin Toxicity." *J.A.M.A.* 245:1939, 1981.

S. H. Powell, "Digoxin Toxicity with Therapeutic Levels." *Drug Intell. Clin. Pharmacol.* 14:547, 1980.

R. E. Rangno, "Propranolol Withdrawal." *Arch. Intern. Med.* 141:161, 1981.

R. A. Remick, et al., "A Case Report of Toxic Psychosis with Low Dose Propranolol Therapy." *Am. J. Psychol.* 138:850, 1981.

M. R. Salzberg, and E. J. Gallagher, "Propranolol Overdose." *Ann. Emergency Med.* 9:26, 1980.

R. F. Tynan, et al., "Self Poisoning with Propranolol." *Med. J. Aust.* 1:82, 1981.

C. Tzen-Wen, H. Tung-Po, and Y. Wu-Chang, "Propranolol Intoxication: Three Case Experiences." *Vet. Hum. Toxicol.* 27:528-530, 1985.

CHAPTER 13 *HEMATINICS: IRON COMPOUNDS*

Hematinics are drugs used in the treatment of anemia to improve the condition of the blood. Iron salts are frequently used alone in the treatment of anemia and in conjunction with vitamins as prophylaxis against iron-deficiency anemia or avitaminosis. Because of these reasons, iron salts are readily available in many homes and are frequently ingested by children. Iron preparations have recently been included under the provisions of the Poison Prevention Packaging Act.

Iron is administered either in ferrous (Fe^{2+}) or ferric (Fe^{3+}) form. The ferric form is reduced by stomach acid to the ferrous, which is then absorbed. The ferrous form is absorbed unchanged. Only a fifth to a third of the amount of iron in iron salts is elemental (Table 13-1), and approximately 10 percent of ingested iron is absorbed when taken in prophylactic or therapeutic doses. However, in massive toxic overdose the normal mucosal block ceases to function and more iron is absorbed. Iron absorption occurs mostly in the upper small intestine.

TABLE 13-1: PERCENTAGE OF ELEMENTAL IRON IN IRON SALTS AVAILABLE OVER-THE-COUNTER

20% of ferrous sulfate	30% of ferrous sulfate, dried
12% of ferrous gluconate	33% of ferrous fumarate
37% of ferric phosphate	12% of ferric pyrophosphate
12% of ferrocholinate	16% of ferroglycine sulfate
48% of ferrous carbonate, anhydrous	

Example: 325 mg of ferrous sulfate contains 65 mg of elemental iron:
325 mg X 0.2(20%) = 65 mg

The daily iron requirement for infants is greater than for older children and adults, but it is only 1 mg of elemental iron/kg/day. The therapeutic dose of iron is higher, approximately 5 to 6 mg of elemental iron/kg/ day. The fatal dose is usually massive, 200 to 300/kg, but it is not an uncommonly ingested dose, since iron tablets "look like candy."

The mechanism of the toxic effect of iron has not been well elucidated, but probably large amounts of iron overcome the normal mucosal block to absorption of iron. Subsequently ferritin, the iron protein compound that is stored intracellularly, escapes into circulation, producing circulatory collapse. Ferritin is a vasodilator.

Poisoning

Acute poisoning. Iron toxicity after large overdose can be divided into three major phases — hemorrhages and gastroenteritis, asymptomatic period, and cardiovascular collapse. Two other sequelae of acute iron intoxication are hepatic damage and pyloric stenosis.

The first phase occurs between 30 minutes and a few hours after ingestion. It is due to the direct corrosive action of the iron salts on the gastrointestinal mucosa, producing a hemorrhagic gastroenteritis characterized by vomiting, hematemesis, abdominal pain, and diarrhea. Dehydration and acidosis may occur, depending on the severity of the intoxication. Excessive blood loss is seldom a problem. A delayed sequela of the described phase is gastrointestinal obstruction due to scarring, which is most significant in the pylorus and leads to pyloric stenosis.

The second phase is apparent recovery and well-being, lasting several hours. Subsequently, the third phase of cardiovascular collapse follows. This third phase occurs 1 to 2 days later and is characterized by shock, convulsion, and death. The third phase is due to the vasodilator properties of ferritin, which leak into the circulation in massive iron overdose.

Severe liver damage in patients who survive the three major phases of acute iron intoxication has been reported. Following intensive and aggressive care numerous patients have survived the initial stages of poisoning only to succumb to the late hepatic toxicity of iron. Renal and pancreatic malfunction may also complicate the clinical picture of these acutely iron-intoxicated patients. Finally, if severely poisoned patients survive, the delayed result of iron intoxication, gastrointestinal obstruction which is most commonly pyloric, can occur.

Chronic poisoning. Chronic iron overload is either idiopathic or occurs because of some underlying illness such as thalassemia that requires frequent blood transfusion.

The nomenclature regarding chronic iron toxicity is confusing, but probably the most accepted terms are *hemochromatosis* for iron deposition in organs such as the liver and pancreas accompanied by *fibrosis* and *hemosiderosis* for iron deposition in these organs without fibrosis. It is well accepted that hemochromatosis leads to hepatic cirrhosis and diabetes mellitus accompanied by a bronze skin color.

Treatment

In managing iron overdoses, first determine the presence or absence of free iron. The only current reliable way to do so is from serum iron and total iron-binding capacity (TIBC). If serum iron exceeds iron-binding capacity, then free serum iron is present. The free serum iron is responsible for cellular toxicity. Iron over 500 micrograms/100 ml is generally toxic and will exceed the iron-binding capacity of most patients at that level.

Institute emergency measures to eliminate the iron tablets from the gastrointestinal tract (see Chap. 2). The use of oral deferoxamine (Desferal), an iron chelating agent, for gastric lavage is controversial. Use sodium bicarbonate (2% to 5% dilution) or sodium phosphate-sodium biphosphate mixture (half-strength Fleet enema) to lavage iron-intoxicated patients, because with iron these compounds form an insoluble salt. At the end of lavage, leave 50 ml of the sodium bicarbonate or phosphate solution in the stomach. When no iron tablets are recovered by either lavage or emesis, take an abdominal x-ray film, since some iron tablets are radiopaque. In one reported case, all the iron tablets matted into a ball that had to be surgically removed. Radiopacity may be used to confirm the ingestion of iron tablets but should not be relied on to rule out an ingestion since radiopacity is related not only to density, but also relative contrast to surrounding tissues and compactness of the pharmaceutical dosage form.

The major chelating agent in the treatment of iron intoxication is deferoxamine. It can be administered orally to decrease the absorption of iron, but this is controversial. The amount of deferoxamine that must be given by mouth or intubation is impractical, and therefore oral administration is not common. Give it when necessary either intravenously or intramuscularly to chelate iron already absorbed. Deferoxamine's value in chronic iron intoxication remains debatable but is undisputed in acute overdose. Deferoxamine is contraindicated in patients with severe renal disease. Both iron salts and deferoxamine can induce hypotension; thus carefully monitor the blood pressure of patients intoxicated with iron who are treated with deferoxamine. Exchange transfusion has been shown to be effective in diminishing circulating iron in acute iron toxicity. If the patient is in shock, start intravenous deferoxamine at a dose of 1 g at an infusion rate not to exceed 15 mg/kg/hr (e.g., give a 10-kg child an initial dose of 150 mg/kg/hr over 6.6 hours to achieve an initial 1-g dose). Subsequent doses of 0.5 g can be administered at the same rate depending on response every 4 to 12 hours. Do not exceed 6 g in 24 hours. If the patient is not in shock, give deferoxamine intramuscularly at a dose of 90 mg/kg up to a maximum single dose of 1 g every 8 hours for 3 doses if serum iron is in excess of TIBC or exceeds 500 micrograms/ml. Manufacturer's recommended dose is 1 g initially followed by 0.5 g every 4 hours for 2 doses. Depending on clinical response, administer subsequent doses of 0.5 g every 4 to 12 hours, not exceeding 6 g in 24 hours. Once a dose of deferoxamine has been given, subsequent serum iron levels will be falsely negative; monitor urine for the characteristic red color indicating chelated complex is being excreted.

References — Chapter 13

M. Barry, "Progress Report: Iron and the Liver." *Gut* 15:324-326, 1974.

D. S. Fischer, R. Parkman, and S. C. Finch, "Acute Iron Poisoning in Children: The Problem of Appropriate Therapy." *J.A.M.A.* 218:1179-1184, 1971.

J. A. James, "Acute Iron Poisoning: Assessment of Severity and Prognosis." *J. Pediatr.* 77:117-119, 1970.

P. G. LaCouture, et al., "Emergency Assessment of Severity of Iron Overdose by Clinical and Laboratory Methods." *J. Pediatr.* 99:89-95, 1981.

N. Movassaghi, G. G. Purugganan, and L. Sunford, "Comparison of Exchange Transfusion and Deferoxamine in the Treatment of Acute Iron Poisoning." *J. Pediat.* 75:604-607, 1969.

T. Peters, et al., "A Simple and Crude Method for the Determination of Serum Iron." *Clin. Med.* 48:280-288, 1956.

W. O. Robertson, "Treatment of Acute Iron Poisoning." *Mod. Treat.* 8:552-560, 1971.

Symposium, "Iron Poisoning." *Clin. Toxicol.* 4:525-642, 1971.

A. Vuthibhagdee, and N. F. Harris, "Antral Stricture as a Delayed Complication of Iron Intoxication." *Radiology* 103:163-164, 1972.

HOUSEHOLD POISONS

The number of chemicals to which one is exposed in the modern household is staggering even if one considers only the number of ready-to-use products available, not to mention a count by ingredients. The kitchen and bathroom with their cleaning and disinfecting agents, the garage and workroom with chemical "tools," cosmetic and personal care products, garden and lawn chemicals, and the almost innumerable ways in which foods can become adulterated tempt one to believe that poisoning is practically inevitable at some time in the home. Exposure to poisonous plants and to bites and stings from venomous animals add to the numerous misadventures that can occur in the home setting.

Children under 5 years of age are particularly at risk of poisoning from the products mentioned above and require constant adult supervision and intervention to prevent poisoning. The next few chapters discuss the most common "household poisonings" and their symptoms and medical management.

CHAPTER 14 *PESTICIDES*

Pesticides or economic poisons are chemicals and materials used to combat pests including microorganisms that afflict animals and plants. In a broader sense pesticides can be defined as all chemicals and materials that by their special, and sometimes selective, poisonous properties are used to safeguard the health, food supply, and property of human beings. Ideally, pesticides should be selective; that is, they should destroy or eliminate the intended pest while having little or no effect on the host. Unfortunately, most pesticides do not have this high degree of selectivity, and a number of clinical intoxications continue to occur, usually as the result of accidents or incorrect methods of distribution and application. The average annual death rate due to pesticides in the United States is estimated by the Public Health Service to be one per 1 million population. Nonfatal reported poisonings approximate one per 10,000 population each year.

Pesticides can be classified according to chemical structure and pharmacotoxicologic properties. This chapter discusses the principal pesticides: insecticides such as the chlorinated hydrocarbons, organophosphates, and carbamates; rodenticides such as warfarin; and certain miscellaneous pesticides.

ORGANOCHLORINE (CHLORINATED HYDROCARBON) INSECTICIDES

Chlorophenothane (DDT) was first synthesized in 1874, but its insecticidal properties were not discovered until 1939. DDT revolutionized the control of insect pests, and other analogs soon followed and led to the proliferation of new synthetic insecticides. As is often the case in a discussion of organic substances, terminology can be confusing. These compounds are not the same as the organochlorine pesticides used as fumigants nor the chlorinated organophosphates, which are discussed later.

The three major kinds of chlorinated hydrocarbon insecticides are DDT analogs, benzene hexachloride (BHC) isomers, and cyclodiene compounds. Chemical structure and activity vary among compounds.

Poisoning

The toxicity described here for the entire group is based largely on DDT but is applicable to all chlorinated hydrocarbon insecticides. Although their mechanism of action in mammals and insects has never been clearly understood, it is apparent that they are neurologic poisons. They are fat-soluble compounds. Numerous studies have undertaken the measurement of levels of chlorinated hydrocarbon insecticides in normal human tissues.

In both acute and chronic poisoning, laboratory techniques can be used to identify halogenated hydrocarbons and their metabolites in blood, urine, gastric contents, and body fat. However, these assays do not correlate well with clinical symptoms. Although these laboratory determinations are sophisticated laboratory procedures, they have limited applicability in emergencies.

Acute poisoning. Acute poisoning brings on marked hyperkinesis with vomiting shortly after ingestion, muscular spasms, ataxia, and fasciculations that usually precede the onset of convulsions. However, high levels of absorption accelerate the onset of many symptoms, and seizure and coma may occur rapidly. Manifestations of central nervous system stimulation from slight exposure include headache, anorexia, nausea, and instability with increasing intensity of exposure. Weakness, paresthesias, tremors, and muscle fibrillation may be observed. Paresthesias of the tongue, face, and lips have been noted early in the course of DDT poisoning, and in severe cases paresthesias may occur in the extremities as well.

Ingestion of large quantities of the dry powder and smaller amounts in organic liquid solvents usually produces symptoms within 1 or 2 hours. In most overexposure situations, symptoms appear within several hours. Although a delay in symptoms of more than 8 hours is unusual in most exposures, it may occur in patients ingesting small amounts of nonsolvent dry preparations.

Chronic poisoning. Chronic toxicity from nonindustrial exposure is a subject of debate and has led to the banning of DDT. Continued low-level exposure does not produce much acute toxicity. Clinical phenomena are similar to those in acute poisoning due to an intense single exposure. However, these agents persist in the environment for long periods and have been implicated as the cause of numerous chronic effects including genetic and carcinogenic mutations as well as bone marrow depression.

Treatment

No specific antidotes exist for chlorinated hydrocarbon pesticide poisoning. Treatment is symptomatic and supportive. Decontamination *must* be carried out as soon as possible. If the insecticide has been ingested, emesis or gastric lavage takes priority. If the patient is wearing contaminated clothing, remove it as soon as possible. Most chlorinated hydrocarbons are absorbed through the skin, and at least one member of the class, dieldrin, can be absorbed easily in this manner from a dry state (i.e., without being a solution). After contaminated clothing is removed, wash away material on the skin, in the hair, and under the nails with water and soap. Petroleum-based solvents present the additional hazard of aspiration pneumonia. With ingestion of large amounts of the highly toxic members of this class of insecticide, aspiration pneumonia is of less significance than the probable systemic effects from ingestion. The reverse may be true when ingestion of a small quantity of a highly diluted solvent is accompanied by coughing. For severe symptoms, use diazepam to control convulsions. Use supportive ventilatory procedures if needed.

Mild intoxication with signs of central nervous system stimulation may be treated with oral barbiturates or diazepam. Symptoms of chlorinated hydrocarbon poisoning may persist as long as a week, and control of symptoms may be necessary for this entire period.

ORGANOPHOSPHORUS INSECTICIDES

The discovery of the insecticidal properties of DDT led to the proliferation of new synthetic chlorinated hydrocarbons. The second massive introduction of new insecticides was initiated by German workers who pioneered in the chemistry and uses of organophosphorus insecticides. These substances were originally developed as chemical warfare agents. Their action in both insects and vertebrates is based on their inactivation of acetylcholinesterase. In human beings a reduction of red blood cell cholinesterase to 25 percent or less of laboratory control indicates significant intoxication.

Acetylcholine, the natural substrate of the enzyme acetylcholinesterase, is a primary neurohumoral transmitter substance in the nervous system and is necessary for impulse transmission. The normal transmission of an impulse by acetylcholine is followed by rapid hydrolysis of the transmitter by the enzyme and limitation of duration and intensity of the stimulus.

The organophosphorus insecticides form unusually stable compounds with the enzyme acetylcholinesterase, and the phosphorylated enzyme loses its normal function as an esterase. Thus, an accumulation of acetylcholine causes a sustained parasympathetic and neuromuscular end-plate stimulation with increased function and ultimately leads to decreased function with a large accumulation of acetylcholine. In the central nervous system initial stimulation followed by depression also occurs.

Poisoning

Acute poisoning. The clinical effects are those of massive cholinergic stimulation with all or most of the following symptoms:

Abdominal pain	Convulsions	Muscular fasciculation
Anorexia	Diaphoresis	Nausea
Ataxia diarrhea	Paralysis	Pulmonary edema
Areflexia	Dyspnea	Salivation
Accelerated peristalsis	Headache	Urination
Blurred vision	Hyperglycemia	Vomiting
Bradycardia	Lacrimation	Weakness
Bronchial hypersecretion	Miosis	
Bronchospasm	Muscle cramps	

Early mydriasis may be followed by alternation of dilation and constriction of the pupils that finally produces constriction. Mydriasis early in the poisoning is seen more often in children than in adults. Death in cases of heavy exposure is usually related to respiratory collapse, reflecting depression of the respiratory center, weakness of the muscles of respiration, bronchoconstriction, and excessive pulmonary secretions.

Chronic poisoning. The medical literature describes both delayed and chronic toxicity from organophosphate insecticides. Delayed toxicity represents an onset of effects on the central and peripheral nervous systems appearing days to weeks after exposure. Delayed toxicity can occur independently of the effects observed in acute poisoning due to cholinesterase inhibition. It is not treatable with atropine and pralidoxime and is thought to be rare. Chronic toxicity is more controversial and appears to be related to the cholinesterase-inhibiting properties of these chemicals, but over prolonged periods. Both types of toxicity are discussed in more detail below.

Although rare, delayed toxicity resulting from exposure to the organophosphates has been confirmed and discussed in the medical literature for over 30 years. The implications are great because research on these chemicals has been intensive in the United States since World War II. However, even before this time delayed neurotoxicity following exposure to other phosphate esters similar to the ones used as pesticides was described during Prohibition in the United States. A series of poisonings occurred when Jamaica ginger extract ("jake") was contaminated with triorthocresyl phosphate (or TOCP, a chemical used as a gasoline additive but also possessing cholinesterase-inhibiting properties) and consumed by alcoholics. This now classic description of neurotoxicity was dubbed "ginger jake paralysis."

In the 1950s reports began to appear about cases of exposure to the organophosphate pesticides that resembled "ginger jake paralysis." In 1953 it was suggested that the cause of this delayed toxicity was due to a "dying back" of the nerve fiber from a direct effect of the pesticide on nerve cells, referred to as demyelination. Demyelination was demonstrated in animals. Initially, it was believed that this pathologic process occurred as a result of a prolonged reduction of the enzyme cholinesterase, which can occur in both acute and chronic poisoning. Two cases of human poisoning with delayed neurotoxicity following an acute poisoning with the pesticide Mipafox seemed to support this contention. Both patients were research chemists working daily with the manufacture of the pesticide. However, in 1977 a case of delayed neurotoxicity was reported in a healthy man aged 28 years who did not previously experience signs or symptoms of acute poisoning. All the laboratory parameters that are indicators of acute poisoning were normal in this patient. Subsequent case reports have appeared that suggest that the phenomenon of delayed toxicity may not be dose related. Therefore, at present, the cause of delayed injury to nervous tissue remains unclear and apparently idiosyncratic.

For a number of years it has thus been clear that many organophosphorus compounds can produce delayed neurotoxicity in low doses, and there is evidence to show that pretreatment with antidotes does not block this effect. This suggests an entirely different pharmacologic pathway for delayed toxicity as compared to acute and chronic poisoning. A biochemical test has been suggested as a means of predicting this tendency of organophosphates to produce delayed neurotoxicity. The case of delayed neurotoxicity in the man aged 28 mentioned above was diagnosed as typical of Guillain-Barré syndrome reported following exposure to merphos (Folex). Merphos was reported in a 1969 study to cause delayed neurotoxicity in animals. This same study demonstrates that chloropyrifos (Dursban) also produces experimentally induced delayed neurotoxicity in animals 3 to 18 days after exposure.

Neurologic and psychologic deficit in chronic poisoning may be subtle and has been reported to occur in the absence of obvious clinical signs of intoxication. Some of these deficits are slowness of thinking, memory defects, irritability, delayed reaction times, impaired vigilance, reduced concentration, linguistic depression, and anxiety. Many of these findings are subjective and difficult to substantiate. The relationship of these findings to cholinesterase levels has not been established, but electromyographic studies have demonstrated abnormal neuromuscular function in pesticide workers who did not have other detectable evidence of intoxication or lowered blood cholinesterase levels.

Treatment

The cornerstone of treatment of acute poisoning from the organophosphorus compounds is the prompt use of atropine in sufficient doses. Atropine does not influence the inactivation of cholinesterase but, rather, limits the exaggerated muscarinic effects. Therefore, blood levels of the enzyme are not increased with even high doses of atropine. If the poisoning is serious enough to warrant the use of a single dose of atropine, the patient should be maintained and observed for 48 hours. Atropine has no effect on the nicotinic manifestation of acetylcholine at the motor end-plates and consequently does not influence weakness of the respiratory musculature. There is danger of ventricular fibrillation in persons who receive atropine in the presence of hypoxia. A reasonable approach to treating a cyanotic patient is to administer oxygen and artificial ventilation to correct hypoxia before administering atropine. Mild atropine intoxication should be achieved, producing slight tachycardia, dry, flushed skin, and reduction of salivary secretion, and may require very large doses. Severely poisoned patients can be given as much as 40 mg of atropine in a single day without producing overatropinization. Never use atropine prophylactically.

As mentioned earlier, atropine does not affect the inactive phosphorylated enzyme complex. However, specific oximes have been developed to accelerate cholinesterase reactivation. The agent (oxime) available in the United States is pralidoxime, 2-pyridinealdoxime (2-PAM). Current evidence suggests that treatment with both atropine and 2-PAM is more effective than treatment with atropine alone. Thus, the treatment in life-threatening situations is as follows: (1) correct hypoxia with suction and other ventilatory measures and maintain a patent airway, (2) administer atropine intravenously, repeated at 5- to 10-minute intervals, (3) administer 2-PAM intravenously, repeating dose if necessary, (4) decontaminate the skin, the hair, and under the nails with soap and water and decontaminate the eyes with normal saline irrigation, and (5) perform other necessary supportive and symptomatic treatment.

CARBAMATE INSECTICIDES

Carbamate insecticides function similarly to the organophosphorus compounds. The mechanism is thought to be enzymatic carbamylation, a process analogous to phosphorylation, but is not established for certain.

Poisoning

Clinical phenomena reflecting esterase inhibition are the same in acute poisoning from the carbamates as from the organophosphates.

Treatment

Atropine is the drug treatment of choice. The oximes should not be used and in the past have even been contraindicated because the inactivating reaction from carbamates on the esterase is readily reversible and normal enzyme is readily regenerated. However, in a life-threatening situation of carbamate poisoning, the benefits of a protopam trial certainly outweighs the risks. Use atropine in the same manner as for the organophosphorus insecticides.

RODENTICIDES

The rodenticides differ markedly in their chemical nature. Consequently, toxicity in humans varies as well. Numerous compounds have been introduced over the years, ranging from the extremely hazardous sodium fluoroacetate to warfarin, which presents minimal hazard to humans. Arsenic and phosphorus are among the older rodenticides, and their toxicity is discussed elsewhere in this manual (see Chap. 20).

SODIUM FLOUROACETATE

Sodium fluoroacetate is still occasionally used in areas where heavy infestation with rats and other small predators exists. It is employed in dilutions of 1:300 to 1:500 either in solution or as a solid mixture with bait. Chemically it is a colorless and odorless salt.

Poisoning

Usually 30 minutes to 2 hours elapses between ingestion and onset of symptoms. The dangerous single dose in humans is between 0.5 and 2 mg/kg. Apparently a combined effect on the heart and the central nervous system is responsible for death in humans in which cardiac features predominate. In humans the first indication of poisoning is nausea and mental apprehension, generally followed by epileptiform convulsions. Cardiac irregularities may exist, and ventricular fibrillation and death may follow. Children appear to be more subject to cardiac arrest than to ventricular fibrillation.

Treatment

For such a nonspecific poison as sodium fluoroacetate, the treatment is mainly symptomatic. Immediate emesis or gastric lavage and cathartics may be helpful. Single doses of magnesium sulfate, 50 percent given intramuscularly, have been used with success to treat sodium fluoroacetate poisoning in animals.

THALLIUM

Thallium sulfate was formerly used as a rodenticide but has been replaced by safer compounds. Thallium acetate was formerly used as a depilatory in a single dose of 8 mg/kg, but this use was discontinued because of the high incidence of toxic side effects. No deaths have been reported at doses of less than 8 mg/kg, but serious symptoms of poisoning have occurred with doses as low as 4 mg/kg of thallium sulfate. The sulfate and acetate salts are equivalent in toxicity.

Poisoning

Acute poisoning. The clinical picture resembles arsenic intoxication.

Signs and symptoms are related to the gastrointestinal tract and the nervous system. Large single doses produce severe gastritis. There may be a delay of up to 5 days before neurologic symptoms appear. Gastrointestinal symptoms include severe paroxysmal abdominal pain, vomiting, diarrhea, anorexia, stomatitis, salivation, and weight loss. Neurologic symptoms range from paresthesias and headache to convulsions and coma.

Chronic poisoning. With continued administration of small doses, symptoms may first be apparent in about a week and progress for several weeks. Symptoms can be nonspecific, and thallium intoxication may not be suspected until depilation occurs.

Treatment

Treat acute poisoning by initiating emesis or gastric lavage. British anti-lewisite (BAL) may be useful as a chelating agent, but clinical evidence of its efficacy is lacking. Another chelating agent, dithizon (diphenylthiocarbazone), has been used with success in treating children severely ill from thallium; however, it is not available as an approved drug for use in human beings.

WARFARIN

Warfarin, 3-(alpha-acetonylbenzyl)-4-hydroxycoumarin (D-Con), and pindone, 3-pivalyl-1, 3 indanedione (Pival), brodifacoum (Talon, Havoc), and diphacinone (Diphacin, Ramik) are currently widely used in rodenticides. They are chemically dissimilar, but their effects on the production of prothrombin in animals are essentially identical, and it is therefore convenient to discuss them together.

Each compound is used at a final concentration dependent on its relative potency (Table 14-1). Rodenticides are frequently distributed in food considered attractive to rats and mice (e.g., cornmeal or peanuts). Specially prepared concentrates for industrial use are also available.

TABLE 14-1: WARFARIN COMPOUNDS

PRODUCTS:	1 mg warfarin or equivalent	15-25 mg (Substantial ingestion)	>than 25 mg (Large ingestion)
warfarin (D-Con Ready Mix) 0.025%	4 gm	60-100 gm	>than 100 gm
warfarin (D-Con Concentrate) 0.3%	0.33 gm	5-8 gm	>than 8 gm
brodifacoum (Talon, Havoc) 0.005%	0.5 gm	7.5-12.5 gm	>than 12.5 gm
Diphacinone (Diphacin) 0.005%	6.7 gm	100-168 gm	>than 168 gm
Pindone (Pival)	1 mg	15-25 mg	>than 25 mg

Warfarin and pindone are dangerous to all mammals and birds, but the hazard is limited to large animals and to humans, since a very large single dose or a number of small doses are necessary to induce characteristic effects.

These compounds inhibit the production of prothrombin, which causes eventual decline of prothrombin levels in the blood. They also damage the integrity of capillary walls. Without prothrombin, hemorrhages are unchecked by clotting, and weakened capillary walls rupture at the slightest injury, making hemorrhages virtually a certainty. Warfarin is not significantly absorbed through the skin. Safety factors and experience with this drug over the years make poisoning in therapeutic doses an unlikely situation.

Poisoning

Acute poisoning. Acute poisoning from a single orally ingested dose is almost unknown. Even single intravenous therapeutic doses usually require up to 14 hours to produce a substantial decrease in prothrombin time. In one reported instance, with a daily ingestion of 1.7 mg/kg/day (equivalent to 1 lb of bait of 0.025 percent warfarin) for 6 consecutive days in an attempted suicide, initial symptoms were back pain and abdominal pain. Onset of symptoms occurred 1 day after the sixth daily dose. A day after onset of symptoms, vomiting and attacks of nosebleed occurred. All the behavioral effects of warfarin and pindone rodenticides are associated with hemorrhage and loss of blood. Hemorrhage may take place in the gastrointestinal tract and be evidenced by vomiting substantial amounts of blood or by blood being passed as feces. The clinical picture consists of rapidly developing weakness and respiratory difficulty as the anemia develops. Hematomas are very common and may occur in any part of the body — subcutaneously, intramuscularly, and in any other area served by capillary beds, particularly the brain.

Treatment

The child who eats a few mouthfuls of warfarin rat bait or any amount less than 15 mg total warfarin equivalent at a single setting is generally not at risk and no treatment is necessary. If larger doses are involved, immediately take blood for prothrombin and other differential diagnostic tests if poisoning from these substances is suspected. If very large amounts are ingested as a single dose, emesis would seem to be a safe precaution even though the dose may not be large enough to produce any clinical symptoms. Give a vitamin K analog at 1 to 5 mg for a child and 10 mg for an adult intramuscularly or orally if the patient is not vomiting. Use activated charcoal and cathartics if large single amounts have been ingested. Treat severe toxicity with intravenous vitamin K in amounts corresponding to laboratory values. Follow the patient's progress by determining prothrombin time; test at least twice daily until a return to normal is clearly established.

MISCELLANEOUS PESTICIDES AND HERBICIDES

Pyrethrum extract from the powdered flowers of several species of chrysanthemum is used in many insect sprays and powders when a rapid knockout effect is required. Many aerosol bombs contain pyrethrum or a pyrethrin. Allethrin is another botanical extract related to pyrethrum and of similar toxicity. Both materials are moderately potent skin sensitizers and cross react with the chrysanthemum, shasta daisy, and ragweed, since they are plant derivatives. Rotenone is also a plant derivative with properties similar to pyrethrum. Nicotine sulfate is a potent neurologic poison that can be absorbed through the skin, in the lungs, and in the gastrointestinal tract. Piperonyl butoxide is not used as an insecticide but as a synergist in combination with insecticides such as pyrethrum, thereby permitting concentrations to be reduced to no more than 10 percent of that otherwise required. It is thought to be comparatively nontoxic.

Arsenicals, for example, Paris green and other inorganic compounds of arsenic, are used with decreasing frequency. Hydrogen cyanide and methyl bromide are used in warehouses and on ships as fumigants.

Larvae of mites and other parasites inhabit the soil, as do various insects, and all are controlled by soil fumigants. The best known of these agents is DD, a mixture of 1,2-dichloropropane and 1,3-dichloropropene, which is an intense irritant of the eyes, skin, and mucosa of the respiratory tract. Other nematocides include methyl bromide, ethyl bromide, and carbamates.

Chlorobenzilate and chlorbenside resemble the chlorinated hydrocarbons and are used as miticides and acaricides. Mammalian toxicity for these agents is not great. Dinitrophenol is a miticide and herbicide of greater toxicity than the two previously mentioned agents.

Herbicides are used to destroy noxious plants. One might expect that herbicides would present less of a hazard to vertebrates, since plants differ markedly from animals in their morphology and physiology. In some instances this is true, but even among the herbicides are highly toxic compounds that have been responsible for fatal poisonings.

Among the more toxic herbicides for humans are the dinitrophenols (also employed as miticides, as previously mentioned). They induce an exaggerated metabolism that can be mistaken for organophosphorus poisoning; take care to avoid misdiagnosis, since atropine is *absolutely contraindicated* in poisoning by dinitrophenolic compounds. The bipyridyl compounds are also toxic for animals, and all species showing similar fatal pulmonary responses after single large doses of paraquat, and hyperexcitability and convulsions following ingestion of Diquat.

More selective weed killers include hydrocarbons such as the chlorinated phenoxyacetic acids (2,4-D and 2,4,5-T) and their salts and esters. These are the most familiar compounds used in homes and gardens and by agencies along highways and roads to control broad-leafed weeds and woody plants. They kill plants by inhibiting plant growth. Animals that have died from massive doses of 2,4-D apparently died of ventricular fibrillation.

Pentachlorophenol is a weed killer, wood preservative, and fungicidal agent often used in building construction. Toxicity from pentachlorophenol (often called "penta") resembles that produced by the nitrophenolic herbicides just discussed, that is, marked increase in the metabolic rate as the result of uncoupling of oxidative phosphorylation. It is readily absorbed through the skin, and quantities absorbed by this route have produced at least two fatalities.

The carbamate herbicides have relatively low acute toxicity, as do the substituted ureas and the triazine herbicides. Animal LD_{50} values for these agents are generally greater than 1,000 mg/kg.

References — Chapter 14

American Public Health Association. "Safe Use of Pesticides." (American Public Health Association Press, 1968).

P. L. Bidstrupp, J. A. Bonnell, and A. G. Beckett, "Paralysis Following Poisoning by a New Organic Phosphorus Insecticide (Mipafox)." *Br. Med. J.* 1:1068, 1953.

F. H. Bledso, and E. Q. Seymour, "Acute Pulmonary Edema Associated with Parathion Poisoning," *Radiology* 103:53-56, 1972.

L. A. Carlson, and B. Kolmodin-Hedman, "Hyperlipoproteinemia in Men Exposed to Chlorinated Hydrocarbon Pesticides." *Acta Med. Scand.* 192:29-32, 1972.

A. H. Conney, et al., "Effects of Environmental Chemicals on the Metabolism of Drugs, Carcinogens and Normal Body Constituents in Man." *Ann. N. Y. Acad. Sci.* 179:155-172, 1971.

J. E. Davies, J. B. Mann, and P. M. Tocci, "Renal Tubular Dysfunction and Amino Acid Disturbances under Conditions of Pesticides Exposure." *Ann. N. Y. Acad. Sci.* 160:323-333, 1969.

C. A. Edwards, "Persistant Pesticides in the Environment." (Cleveland, OH: Chemical Rubber Publishing Company, 1970).

H. K. Fisher, M. Humphries, and R. Bails, "Paraquat Poisoning: Recovery from Renal and Pulmonary Damage." *Ann. Intern. Med.* 75:731-736, 1971.

A. Hamilton, and H. L. Hardy, "Industrial Toxicology." (Acton, MA: Publishing Science Group, 1974).

R. M. Hasan, et al., "Correlation of Serum Pseudocholinesterase and Clinical Course in Two Patients Poisoned with Organophosphate Insecticide." *Clin. Toxicol.* 18:401-407, 1981.

W. J. Hayes, *Clinical Handbook on Economic Poisons.* U. S. Public Health Service Publication No. 476. (Washington, DC: U.S. Government Printing Office, 1963).

K. W. Jager, *Aldrin, Dieldrin, Endrin and Telodrin.* (Amsterdam: Elsevier Publishing Company, 1970).

M. Krogen, "Insecticide Residues in Human Milk." *J. Pediatr.* 80:401-405, 1972.

F. S. Lisella, K. R. Long, and H. G. Scott, "Toxicology of Rodenticides and Their Relation to Human Health." *J. Environ. Health* 33:231-237, 361-365, 1971.

J. D. G. Malone, et al., "Paraquat Poisoning: A Review of 19 Cases." *J. Irish Med.* A. 64:59-68, 1971.

W. J. Hayes, Jr. "Studies on Exposure During the Use of Anti-Cholinesterase Pesticides." *Bull. WHO* 44:277-288, 1971.

F. Matsamura, "Toxicology of Insecticides." (New York: Plenum Press, 1975).

B. J. McDonagh, and J. Martin, "Paraquat Poisoning in Children." *Arch. Dis. Child.* 45:425-427, 1970.

K. N. P. Mickleson, and D. B. Fulton, "Paraquat Poisoning Treated by a Replacement Blood Transfusion: Case Report." *N. Z. Med. J.* 74:26-27, 1971.

T. H. Milby, "Prevention and Management of Organophosphate Poisoning." *J.A.M.A.* 216:2131-2133, 1971.

T. Namba, "Cholinesterase Inhibition by Organophosphorus Compounds and Its Clinical Effects." *Bull. WHO* 44:289-307, 1971.

T. Namba, et al., "Poisoning Due to Organophosphate Insecticides." *Am. J. Med.* 50:475-492, 1971.

D. L. Nelson, "Organophosphorus Compounds: The Past and the Future." *Clin. Toxicol.* 5:223-230, 1972.

W. M. Sare, "Chronic Poisoning by a Phosphate Ester Insecticide, Malathion." *N. Z. Med. J.* 75:93-94, 1972.

M. K. J. Siddiqui, et al., "Long Term Occupational Exposure to DDT." *Intern. Arch. Occup. Environ. Health* 48:301-304, 1981.

U. S. Department of Interior Publication No. 84., *Handbook of Toxicity of Pesticides to Wildlife.* (Washington, DC: U.S. Government Printing Office, 1970).

J. Willems, P. Vermiere, and G. Rolly, "Some Observations on Severe Human Poisonings with Organophosphorus Pesticides." *Arch. Toxicol.* 28:182-191, 1971.

A. Zavon, "Treatment of Organophosphorus and Chlorinated Hydrocarbon Intoxications." *Mod. Treat.* 8:503-510, 1971.

CHAPTER 15 *HYDROCARBONS*

The simplest of organic compounds containing only hydrogen and carbon are called hydrocarbons. Those derived from mineral sources find most of their application in industrialized societies where they are ubiquitous as solvents, dry cleaning fluids, gasolines, spot removers, kerosene, lighter and starter fluids, and mineral seal oil in polishes and waxes, to name only a few of their uses. In addition, certain plants on distillation yield what are known as volatile or essential oils. A few of these volatile oils (e.g., turpentine and pine oil), contain high percentages of hydrocarbons.

Whether their origin is petroleum or plants, chemical composition of all hydrocarbons is similar and allows their consideration as toxic agents to be based on a structural classification (see also Chap. 22).

ALIPHATIC HYDROCARBONS

The aliphatic hydrocarbons include the saturated (paraffin or alkane) and the unsaturated (olefin or alkene) compounds, which are derived almost exclusively from petroleum or petroleum processing. Compounds in the aliphatic series are used as fuels, solvents, and lubricants. Depending on the length of the carbon chain, they exist either as gases (methane, ethane, propane, and butane), as liquids in the pentane series, C5 through C16, or as solids when they contain more than 16 carbon atoms.

From the toxicologic standpoint these compounds are not particularly active. The first two members of the series, methane and ethane, have no known biologic properties and exert an effect only as simple asphyxiants. The saturated hydrocarbons from propane through the octanes have increasingly strong narcotic properties. Heavier members of this series are not sufficiently volatile to produce narcotizing concentrations in air unless they are heated or are in a vapor-saturated atmosphere such as that encountered in tanks and other enclosures.

The vapors of compounds from pentane through octane are increasingly irritating to mucous membranes. Exposure to the gases of this series and to most of the solvent mixes is almost entirely limited to industrial exposure. Contact with individual members of the series is rare. Most commonly, exposure is to mixtures that may be variously termed petroleum ether, benzine (not benzene), petroleum naphtha, gasoline, kerosene, mineral spirits, stoddard solvent, and Varsol.

Poisoning

Acute poisoning. In massive acute exposure from inhalation of the concentrated vapors, rapid central nervous system depression and cardiac arrhythmias may occur, with sudden collapse, deep coma, and death. There may be a convulsion indicating brain irritation or apneic anoxia. Full recovery without sequelae is the rule. However, cerebral micro-hemorrhages and focal postinflammatory scarring have been suggested as the etiology of epileptiform seizures months after the acute episode. Irritation of the upper and lower respiratory tract and visceral damage have also been described.

More recently, cases have been described of persons who intentionally inhaled vapors of volatile liquids such as gasoline for kicks. It appears that in these instances death is due to fatal cardiac arrhythmias in which the endogenous release of epinephrine is implicated. In industrial situations, kerosene and other heavier liquids are insufficiently volatile to cause respiratory tract damage. However, these materials most commonly enter the lungs on aspiration following ingestion and cause chemical pneumonia, which usually peaks in 2 to 8 hours and clears in 3 to 5 days if superinfection with bacteria does not occur. Toxic effects of ingested aliphatic hydrocarbons are directly related to complications of aspiration. Aside from minor irritation, these substances are not particularly harmful to the gastrointestinal tract.

When large amounts of low-viscosity mixtures such as gasoline are aspirated, they irritate the lungs and respiratory tract and lead to either rapid death from cardiac arrest, asphyxia or respiratory paralysis, or severe chemical pneumonitis and central nervous system manifestations (e.g., convulsions and coma). Aspiration of small quantities of slightly heavier molecular weight compounds such as kerosene results in a slower progression of events marked by chemical pneumonitis with prominent endothelial damage and pulmonary hemorrhage and edema. Heavier and more viscous materials such as mineral oil and motor oil are not readily aspirated. These high-viscosity oils can produce a chronic localized tissue response termed *lipoid pneumonia*, which is observed in persons who take mineral oil-based nose drops over a number of years.

Chronic poisoning. There is no convincing evidence that prolonged exposure to the vapors of aliphatic hydrocarbons causes permanent harmful effects. Chronic permanent effects such as bone marrow depression are probably due to aromatic contaminants.

For workers who are repreatedly exposed to the gases and very volatile liquids in this series, threshold limit values (TLV) have been established. Exposure to excessive levels usually produces acute symptoms such as exhilaration, dizziness, and headache, which serve as a warning. There may be a loss of appetite, nausea, persisting taste of gasoline, confusion, inability to do fine work, and, in extreme cases, loss of consciousness.

Solvents in this classification are all primary irritants and defatting agents when applied to the skin. As fat solvents they extract sebum from the skin, leaving a dry, irritated surface prone to cracking and bacterial infection. Prolonged exposure without the use of protective clothing should be avoided.

Treatment

In acute inhalation, removing the overcome victim from the contaminated area usually results in rapid clearing of symptoms (see Chap. 2).

Following ingestion, the patient may appear only mildly symptomatic or asymptomatic. It has been suggested that ingested quantities greater than 1 ml/kg of these straight chain hydrocarbons may produce central nervous system depression. If this quantity can be documented from the history, some people recommend emesis or lavage before symptoms can occur. Although emesis is controversial, it appears to be the safest and most effective means of removing large amounts of hydrocarbons from the stomach of a conscious patient. Reserve gastric lavage for a comatose patient (see Chap. 2). However, emesis is usually only indicated when the hydrocarbon also contains heavy metals, insecticides, or other toxic substances. Children who ingest a taste or a mouthful of a pure hydrocarbon do not require emesis. Aspiration of even small amounts must be ruled out and is of particular importance when some of the more volatile distillates such as naphtha are the poisoning agents. Dyspnea or tachypnea, cyanosis with rales, rhonchi, and dull and diminished breath sounds at the base of one or both lungs may indicate aspiration. Fever and tachycardia may also be present. If pulmonary signs are present, oxygen is the most valuable agent to relieve respiratory distress and anoxia. Activated charcoal may be of value but is not generally recommended. If central nervous system depression does occur, the treatment is entirely symptomatic and supportive. Secondary bacterial infection is treated with antibiotics, but these should probably not be used prophylactically. Corticosteroids have been shown to be of no value in resolving hydrocarbon pneumonitis. Extracorporeal membrane oxygenation is a procedure that has demonstrated success in treating cases of massive hydrocarbon aspiration. However, this technique is not available at all medical facilities.

AROMATIC HYDROCARBONS

The aromatic series of hydrocarbons is based on benzene molecules, which incorporate one or more benzene rings and are thus unsaturated cyclic structures. They can correctly be referred to as petroleum distillates, since at present the petrochemical industry provides the major source of aromatic compounds. Both coal- and petroleum-derived aromatics are produced in ways that lead to complicated mixtures of many compounds in the series.

Benzene is the parent member of this series and the most significant toxicologically. Do not confuse it with benzine, which denotes the low-boiling petroleum fraction of mostly aliphatic compounds and is similar to ordinary gasoline. Benzene is an important solvent used for laboratory extraction and chromatographic separation but is used mostly in the synthesis of other organic compounds such as styrene, phenol, and nylon intermediates.

Toluene and xylene are used as industrial solvent mixtures. They are less volatile than benzene. Diphenyl and diphenyloxide are used in industry primarily as heat transfer media. Diphenyl is also used as a fungistatic agent to preserve fruit. Naphthalene, familiar as mothballs (now largely replaced by paradichlorobenzene), is used as a chemical intermediate in the production of phthalic acid and derivatives for the dye and plastic industries.

Poisoning

Acute poisoning. Like most organic solvents, benzene is a central nervous system depressant at high concentrations, but violent excitement and delirium may precede unconsciousness. Essentially the same symptoms follow both ingestion of the liquid and inhalation of the vapor. Industrial exposure to toxic levels of benzene vapor may bring on mild manifestations such as lightheadedness and headache, which can progress to respiratory paralysis and death. The pattern of apparent drunken behavior due to benzene is referred to as a "benzol jag" and consists of euphoria, unsteady gait, and confusion. Recovery from acute benzene narcosis is complete unless the levels and duration of exposure cause pathologic changes. As with other hydrocarbons, give the usual attention to ingestions accompanied by coughing, choking, dyspnea, and cyanosis for the possibility of aspiration. The aromatic hydrocarbons present a greater danger by ingestion inasmuch as they are more readily absorbed in the gastrointestinal tract. Treat ingestion of even small quantities of aromatic hydrocarbons, especially benzene, as an emergency. When ingested, these fat-soluble solvents produce a burning sensation in the mouth and stomach and may induce nausea, salivation, and vomiting. These agents are claimed to sensitize the myocardium to epinephrine, producing cardiac arrhythmias. Acute exposure to large amounts of benzene can also cause hematopoietic changes, which may appear long after the initial exposure. Xylene and toluene are less toxic to bone marrow and differ from benzene in that survival from acute single exposure appears to produce almost no residual effects.

Chronic poisoning. Chronic poisoning from the aromatic series of hydrocarbons is of greater toxicologic significance. It is an industrial problem that has lessened over the years with improvement in industrial hygiene. Benzene is the most toxic of the group. Unfortunately, the toxic manifestations of benzene poisoning are insidious at onset, and a case may be well advanced at the time of diagnosis. Common initial findings are nonspecific and may include fatigue and loss of appetite. Hematologic evaluation may show anemia, leukopenia, and thrombocytopenia. However, all three cell lines are not always affected or affected to the same degree. Immature cells may be found in the peripheral blood, and there may be eosinophilia or leukocytosis. The bone marrow may be hypoplastic, hyperplastic, or relatively unchanged. These observations do not correlate well with the clinical picture, the character of the exposure, or the prognosis. In some workers with chronic benzene poisoning, there is evidence for shortened red cell survival and extramedullary hematopoiesis. Clinically, idiopathic aplastic anemia and bone marrow failure due to benzene cannot be distinguished. Benzene has also been implicated as the etiologic agent producing some forms of leukemia that appear without an antecedent history of aplastic anemia. Thus, hematotoxic disorders can develop in persons soon after exposure or after periods of 20 to 30 years without exposure to benzene. Chromosomal genetic differences have been suggested as a possible factor in the range of response in persons exposed to benzene.

Toluene and xylene have been implicated along with benzene in producing injury to the hematopoietic system. However, close examination usually reveals the presence of significant amounts of benzene in solvent mixtures derived from coal tar distillation. In some occurrences of aplastic anemia when exposure to benzene-free toluene was established, the history revealed prior exposure to benzene. Isolated instances of bone marrow injury and a history of exposure to agents other than benzene necessitate viewing injuries by toluene and xylene with caution. A number of nonspecific symptoms are reported to have occurred on exposure to high concentrations of diphenyl, diphenyl oxide, and naphthalene. The latter agent as a component of mothballs can cause an acute hemolytic anemia associated with accidental ingestion in individuals with a glucose-6-phosphate dehydrogenase deficiency.

Treatment

Treat the acute ingestion of benzene more aggressively than a poisoning involving the aliphatic series. Consider ingestion of any amount a large quantity and begin treatment with emesis and, in an unconscious patient, with gastric lavage. Other aromatic hydrocarbon toxic doses depend on the individual substance. Xylene and toluene are not as poisonous as benzene, but a good range of toxicity following ingestion is not available. Activated charcoal appears to be effective as an adsorptive agent for these cyclic compounds. Handle the possibility of aspiration pneumonia in the same way as described for the aliphatic hydrocarbons (see earlier in this chapter).

Therapy for chronic poisoning, when it is manifested as either aplastic anemia or leukemia, is that used when these diseases occur without known cause.

References — Chapter 15

D. T. Brown, M. Jones, "Mortality and Industrial Hygiene Study of Workers Exposed to Polychlorinated Biphenols." *Arch. Environ. Health* 36:120-126, 1981.

W. D. Collom, and C. L. Winek, "Detection of Glue Constituents in Fatalities Due to 'Glue-Sniffing'." *Clin. Toxicol.* 3:125-130, 1970.

E. G. Gonzalez, and J. A. Downey, "Polyneuropathy in a Glue Sniffer." *Arch. Phys. Med.* 53:333-337, 1972.

E. Press, et al., "Cooperative Kerosene Poisoning Study." *Pediatrics* 29:648-674, 1962.

G. B. Raffi, and P. S. Violante, "Is Freon a Neurotoxin? A Case Report." *Intern. Arch. Occup. Environ. Health* 49:125-130, 1981.

H. C. Shirkey, "Treatment of Petroleum Distillate Ingestion." *Mod. Treat.* 8:580-592, 1971.

R. W. Steele, R. H. Conklin, and H. M. Mark, "Corticosteroids and Antibiotics for the Treatment of Fulminant Hydrocarbon Ingestion." *J.A.M.A.* 219:1434-1437, 1972.

E. C. Vigliani, "Benzene, Chromosome Changes and Leukemia." *J. Occup. Med.* 11:148-149, 1969.

M. S. Wolf, et al., "Human Tissue Burdens of Halogenated Aromatic Chemicals in Michigan." *J.A.M.A.* 247:2112-2115, 1982.

CHAPTER 16

SOAPS, DETERGENTS, CORROSIVES, AND COSMETICS

Toxicologically cleaners and cosmetics are important because they comprise a large percentage of accidental exposures in children every year. A discussion of their toxicity requires an understanding of some basic differences in their preparation and use.

SOAPS AND DETERGENTS

The term *soap* is loosely applied to a variety of cleaning materials, but a true soap is specifically a salt of a fatty acid, usually made by the action of alkali on natural fats and oils or on the fatty acids obtained from animal or vegetable sources. Consumer soap products are usually based on the sodium salt of fatty acids. Soap is one type of surface active agent, or surfactant, and it was the leading surfactant used in household cleaning products until a few years after World War II.

Shortly before World War II, new nonsoap surfactants developed as bases for cleaning products were found to be more efficient than soap in hard water and could be formulated to meet special cleaning needs. These new types of washing products were called *synthetic detergents*, a term that may cause confusion. Strictly speaking, a detergent is anything that cleans, including soap, washing soda, and synthetic compounds. In common usage, however, the term *synthetic detergent* and its contraction, detergent, have come to mean the household cleaning products that are based on nonsoap surfactants and that are primarily used for laundering and dishwashing. Detergents are usually sulfonated or phosphorylated hydrocarbons such as alkylbenzene sulfonate (ABS) and linear alkylate sulfonate (LAS).

Soaps react with minerals in hard water, forming insoluble precipitates known as "soap curd" or "scum." This inherent disadvantage of soaps has limited their use as effective laundering agents, since scum settles on clothes and causes a grayish discoloration. To overcome this property, chemical "builders" can be added, usually inorganic salts, to maintain alkalinization in wash water. These builders are almost universally present in laundry soaps and in synthetic detergents to enhance detergency, to disperse and suspend dirt, and to maintain proper pH of washing solutions. The most commonly used builders are phosphates, silicates, and carbonates. Phosphates, generally sodium tripolyphosphate, are the inorganic ingredients that historically have been used in the largest volume in detergent formulations, particularly in heavy-duty home laundering products. Because of environmental concern, the use of phosphates has been curtailed pending the development of substitutes that are as safe and effective. Consumer demands for detergent products in areas where phosphates are limited or banned are being met by making available low-phosphate and nonphosphate detergent products, some of which contain carbonates and silicates at proportions higher than those typical of analogous phosphate-based products. Soaps described on the label as light duty are unbuilt; heavy-duty soaps contain builders.

Carboxylated soaps have been used for many centuries, but during the early twentieth century (notably during World War I) fat shortages led to the development of synthetic detergents. Surface active agents (surfactants), when properly blended with other organic and inorganic agents, can be formulated to perform many detergent operations better than do carboxylated soaps. Detergents dissolve readily in any water temperature and do not form scum. A dual characteristic of detergents is that the molecule has water-attracting tendencies (hydrophilic) while at the same time possesses chemical groups that are hydrophobic. The surfactants used in detergents are chemically classified as anionic, cationic, and nonionic. In the anionic surfactants the surface activity is due to a negative ion, whereas the reverse is true in cationic material. Nonionic surfactants demonstrate surface activity although they contain neither negative or positive ions. Household detergents are based on anionic and nonionic surfactants.

Poisoning

Acute poisoning. The cationic detergents are without question more toxic than the anionic and the nonionic detergents.

Anionic detergents. The anionic detergents are the most important class of detergents economically. They consist of salts of fatty acids or alcohols and sulfonated and phosphorylated hydrocarbons. One of the most common agents is ABS (alkylbenzene sulfonate). By themselves anionic surfactants have low toxicity, causing mild, local irritation of the skin, eyes, and mucosal tissues. The addition of builders to this class significantly raises the toxicity. The phosphates (e.g., sodium trip-olyphosphate) were heavily used previously to alkalinize but added only slightly to the irritant and emetic effects. The use of silicates and carbonates in low-phosphate products raises the products' alkalinity and increases their irritant qualities. Highly alkaline detergents may even produce severe eye irritation and oral and esophageal burns. Many electric dishwasher detergents typically contain these agents and have a very high degree of alkalinity and should be considered to have toxic effects similar to caustics. In general, the toxicity of liquid detergents is lower than that of powders and granules because of their formulation in aqueous or hydroalcoholic solutions. Additives in detergents such as bleaches, enzymes, and bactericidal agents are usually in low concentration and do not influence a product's toxicity.

An undesirable effect of the ABSs, in contrast to soap and fatty alcohol-based synthetic detergents, is that their high foam is difficult to eliminate. It remains on the surface of waste water as it passes through towns in drains to sewers and sewage systems, then to rivers, and finally to the sea. Foam causes difficulties in river navigation, and because it retards biologic degradation of organic material in sewage, it also causes problems in sewage water regeneration systems. In countries where sewage water is used for irrigation, foam is also a problem. Intensive research in the 1960s led to changes in the alkylbenzene sulfonate molecules. The tetrapropylenes (the alkyl molecular group used in the past obtained from the petrochemical gas propylene), which have a branched structure, were replaced by an alkyl group consisting of straight carbon chains easily broken down by bacteria. The resultant products were the linear alkylate sulfonate (LAS)-based detergents, which are also known as soft or biodegradable detergents. LAS products are slightly less toxic than ABS products but the difference is not of toxicologic significance.

Cationic detergents. Cationic detergents are used in higher concentrations, primarily in industrial and institutional antiseptics and disinfectants and extensively in lesser concentrations in some household agents (e.g., in fabric softeners or pharmaceuticals).

Structurally, cationic detergents are organically synthesized products having as the hydrophobic portion a nitrogen with four attached hydrocarbons (commonly called quaternary ammonium compounds), putting the nitrogen in a positive state.

Unlike the anionic detergents, the cationic detergents when taken internally can result in serious acute systemic toxicity as well as cause local caustic damage in high concentrations (usually greater than 20 percent). Systemic effects may be seen regardless of the concentration if the ingested amount exceeds 1 g of the cationic substance. The symptoms and signs from ingestion are nausea, vomiting, shock, convulsions, and coma as quickly as 1 to 4 hours after ingestion due to rapid absorption. Since they are readily absorbed, these detergents interfere with any cellular functions. The cationic detergents are rapidly inactivated by the tissues they contract.

Nonionic detergents. Nonionic detergents are commonly found in toilet soaps and light-duty laundry and hand dishwashing products. Expect only mild irritation of the skin and mucous membranes. Ingestion causes no systemic effects. Treat gastric irritation, if it occurs at all, with demulcents (e.g., milk).

Some typical nonionic detergents are alkyl aryl polyether sulfates, alcohol sulfonates, alkyl phenol polyglycol ethers, and polyethylene glycol alkyl aryl ethers.

Chronic poisoning. The only chronic problem with detergents seems to be dermatologic. They irritate the skin by removing natural oils, causing redness and soreness (the well-known dermatitis). In sensitive persons they can also cause weeping, cracking, scaling, and blistering.

Treatment

Ingestion of anionic detergents does not constitute a serious problem. Usually, depending on the quantity ingested, only emesis is necessary. However, pay close attention to the formulation of anionic detergents for the possible presence of alkaline corrosives used as builders (discussed earlier). The presence of phosphates, carbonates, or silicates should suggest treatment the same as for any caustic material.

Most cationic detergents, in addition to being rapidly inactivated by body tissues, are also inactivated by soaps (which are anionic). Thus a mild soap solution may be used as an antidote following oral ingestion to neutralize the unabsorbed residual cationic detergent, but it is ineffective against the systemic effects. Ingestions of cationic detergents over 20 percent can produce corrosive burns of the mouth, throat, and esophagus. Perform immediate dilution with a mild soap solution, water, or milk. Ensure an adequate airway. Consider endotracheal intubation or tracheotomy if acute respiratory obstruction occurs following glottic burns. Use general measures for systemic symptoms to support respiration and treat convulsions.

Nonionic detergents require no treatment if ingested in small amounts. Induce emesis if very large amounts have been ingested.

CORROSIVES

Corrosives are agents employed for their strong reactivity or disinfectant properties. Many are strong alkalies, and others are corrosive acids. Traditionally the name *caustic* refers to caustic soda (sodium hydroxide), but as an adjective it refers to any compound chemically similar to sodium hydroxide and any strongly alkaline material that has a corrosive or irritating effect on living tissue. High-percentage ammonia solutions, oven cleaners, and drain cleaners (potassium and sodium hydroxide) are among the most common strongly alkaline cleaning agents. Corrosive acids such as oxalic and sulfuric are also used for various cleaning purposes and are discussed in this chapter.

Poisoning

Although alkalies and acids both destroy tissue, their causative mechanisms differ. Alkaline corrosives, frequently referred to as caustic agents, produce necrosis with fat saponification that is deep and penetrating, often resulting in severe effects such as esophageal perforation. Ingested alkalies cause the deeper burns that are associated with severe scarring and stricture formation. Since these agents react with proteins and fats to form proteinates and soaps, respectively, they produce soft, white burns on contact with human tissue. Skin exposure may produce first- or second-degree burns; third-degree burns are possible depending on the alkali and duration of contact. Sodium hydroxide, or lye, is the most frequent and serious offender. In addition to its saponifying (soap-producing) and protein-solvent properties, lye is markedly hygroscopic, a characteristic that contributes greatly to its penetration of deeper tissue layers, resulting in liquefaction necrosis. The severity of the lesion produced depends on the corrosive agent swallowed (e.g., the just-mentioned hygroscopic tendency of lye), the concentration, the quantity, and the duration of contact with the tissues. A 3.8 percent (1 N) solution of sodium hydroxide applied for 10 seconds to the esophagus will necrose the mucosa, the submucosa, and some of the inner longitudinal muscle fibers, while a 22.5 percent (7 N) solution applied for the same time will extend through the entire esophageal wall and affect the periesophageal tissues. Note that granulated household drain cleaners typically have from 8 to 50 percent sodium hydroxide as the chief ingredient, and liquid drain cleaners usually contain 8.5 percent lye (sodium hydroxide).

Injuries of the esophagus due to caustic burns are classified similarly to the classification for thermal burns of the skin: (1) first-degree burns, in which only superficial sloughing of the mucosa occurs, (2) second-degree burns, in which deeper transmucosal tissue damage occurs and all layers of the esophagus are involved, with exudate ulceration, loss of mucosa, and erosion through the esophageal wall into the periesophageal tissues, (3) third-degree burns, in which erosion of the esophageal wall into the periesophageal tissues occurs, including the mediastinum and the pleural or peritoneal cavities.

Liquid drain cleaners, introduced in the United States in 1967, can affect all mucosal surfaces of the upper gastrointestinal tract. Most patients with a history of liquid caustic ingestion are found to have a serious esophageal lesion, and almost all progress to extensive stricture formation.

Acids are used in toilet bowl cleaners, for cleaning metals, and to effect a number of chemical reactions. Corrosive effects are produced whenever the acid comes in contact with tissues such as the mucous membranes, tongue, pharynx, esophagus, stomach, and small intestine. As with alkalies the damage is proportionate to the concentration and duration of exposure, but the injury is usually less penetrating than in an alkali burn. A coagulation necrosis results. The ingestion of as little as 1 ml of a strong acid has caused death.

Corrosive acids destroy tissues by direct chemical action. The tissue protein is converted to acid proteinate, which dissolves in the concentrated acid. Hemoglobin is converted to dark acid hematin and is precipitated, resulting in a dark eschar. The intense stimulation by acid causes reflex loss of vascular tone.

Treatment

In patients who ingest an alkali, never lavage the stomach or induce emesis. Immediate dilution with milk or water is the most important aspect of emergency first aid. Time is crucial in preventing permanent serious damage. Twenty seconds following the instillation of 15 ml of Liquid Plumber into the esophagi of anesthetized dogs a violent to-and-fro or seesaw action between the stomach and esophagus of the gastric contents developed.

Admit all individuals with physical findings indicating caustic ingestion to a hospital. In patients who are hypotensive, insert arterial and central venous catheters for constant pressure monitoring. Treat hypovolemia with either whole blood or colloid-containing fluids. Carefully observe the patient for airway obstruction. Endotracheal intubation or tracheotomy may be needed. Fruit juices and the like for neutralization are of little or no value and may be dangerous.

Administer antibiotics as soon as the diagnosis is established. Perform esophagoscopy no more than 24 hours after ingestion. Steroids and antibiotics are recommended to reduce the incidence of stricture formation.

In acid ingestion, never lavage the stomach or induce emesis. Immediate dilution with milk or water is the most important aspect of emergency first aid. Dilute the ingested acid approximately 100 times to render it harmless to tissue. Analgesics such as morphine sulfate are beneficial but not in a dose that will depress the central nervous system.

Maintain an adequate airway to prevent asphyxia from glottal edema, maintain adequate blood pressure and nutrition, and perform surgical intervention if clinical signs or symptoms of esophageal or gastric perforation exist.

Use antibiotics and systemic corticosteroids to reduce the incidence of esophageal stricture formation. In cases of acid inhalation, corticosteroids may reduce pulmonary fibrosis.

COSMETICS

Cosmetics are preparations intended for application on the skin, hair, and nails to beautify the person. Accidental ingestion of these substances is common. Shampoos, hair-waving and hair-straightening solutions, hair dyes and sprays, depilatories, deodorants, and suntan preparations are a few of the common cosmetics ingested.

Poisoning

Shampoos are either vegetable oils saponified with an alkali (sodium, potassium, or ammonium salts) or synthetic detergents. The danger of toxicity by ingestion is minimal. Dry shampoos, however, can be dangerous because they may contain isopropyl and methyl alcohol.

Hair-waving preparations are alkaline caustics that may contain ammonium hydroxide and potassium carbonate or bicarbonate. These alkalies are neutralized with weak acids such as peroxides and perborates and, in the older preparations, with the very toxic bromates. Present cold hair-waving products contain alkaline salts of thioglycolic acid, which are strongly irritating but not very caustic. Hair-straightening solutions are similar to hair-waving preparations. The new ones are thioglycolates with a weak solution of formalin as a fixative.

Hair dyes can be safe organic vegetable tints such as indigo; toxic metallic preparations containing lead, iron, silver, cobalt, or nickel; or the commonly used synthetic organic oxidation dyes made of aniline, amines, or sulfonated azos. One of the most commonly used dyes is paraphenylenediamine (para dye), containing hydrogen peroxide as the oxidizing agent. The phenylenediamines have strong sensitizing properties and can cause severe direct eye and skin irritation and probably bladder carcinoma. A common contaminant of the para dyes, beta-naphthylamine, produces bladder carcinoma.

Hair sprays contain natural and synthetic resins such as polyvinylpyrrolidone. When inhaled, hair sprays produce thesaurosis, pulmonary granulomatosis consisting of hilar lymphadenopathy and diffuse pulmonary infiltration.

Depilatory agents are usually soluble sulfides (barium and sodium) or calcium thioglycolates. They irritate the skin and, when ingested, the gastrointestinal tract. Convulsions, hypoglycemia, and respiratory failure may occur with intoxication from a large dose of the sulfides.

Deodorants can be simple antibacterial agents in a cream base or antiperspirant containing salts of aluminum, zinc, zirconium, and so forth. Unless very large quantities are ingested, deodorants cause no ill effect. However, they have strong sensitizing properties, and those containing zirconium salts are no longer available because they produce chronic granulomatous lesions.

Suntan preparations contain several agents such as titanium dioxide and iron oxide in ethyl alcohol. Ingesting these compounds induces acute alcoholic intoxication.

Boric acid and borates are used as antiseptics, preservatives, and fungistatics in cleaning agents and talcum powders. Indiscriminate use of boric acid on broken skin and mucosa produces boric acid poisoning characterized by erythema, exfoliation of the skin ("boiled-lobster appearance"), fever, vomiting, anuria, and convulsions.

Treatment

Fortunately, most cosmetics are not very toxic, but if substantial quantities have been ingested, follow the principles outlined in Chapter 2. With some very toxic ingredients, such as the bromates, more heroic measures to limit the effective dose may be required, such as dialysis. Because of the seemingly infinite number of individual in-gredients, contact the regional poison center, product in hand, to discuss the components of each brand name item.

Supportive care is always essential. For example, dilute with milk when there is gastric irritation and maintain an airway, hydration, and nutrition when indicated.

References — Chapter 16

K. Benirschke, "Time Bomb of Lye Ingestions." (editorial) *Am J. Dis. Child.* 17:135-138, 1981.

L. J. Casarett, and J. Doull, *Toxicology: The Basic Science of Poisons*, 2nd ed. (New York: Macmillan, 1980).

G. C. Chong, et al., "Management of Corrosive Gastritis Due to Ingested Acid." *Mayo Clin. Proc.* 49:861-865, 1974.

M. Gleason, et al., *Clinical Toxicology of Commerical Products.* (Baltimore: Williams & Wilkins, 1969).

L. J. Goldwater, "Mercury in the Environment." *Scientific American,* May 1971.

Haller et al., "Pathophysiology and Management of Acute Corrosive Burns of the Esophagus." *J. Pediatr. Surg.* 6:578-584, 1971.

G. G. Hawley, *The Condensed Chemical Dictionary* (New York: Van Nostrand Reinhold, 1971), p. 674.

M. Hennessy, "Corrosive Esophagitis: Acute Management With a Case Report of Early Surgical Intervention." *Minn. Med.* 52:1661-1663, (Oct) 1969.

R. H. Hoy, "Accidental Systemic Exposure to Sodium Hypochloride (Clorox)." *Am. J. Hosp. Pharmacol.* 38:1512-1515, 1981.

M. M. Kirsh, and F. Ritter, "Caustic Ingestion and Subsequent Damage to the Oropharnygeal and Digestive Passages." *Ann. Thorac. Surg.* 21:74-82, 1976.

L. E. Kotowski, "Serum Sickness Due to Hair Straightener." *Br. Med. J.* 284:470-472, 1982.

CHAPTER 17 *PLANT POISONING*

Most plants are not toxic and are actually used as food sources. Some plants, such as those which produce gastrointestinal irritation, are mildly toxic; a few are extremely toxic. The major toxic principles in plants are alkaloids, polypeptides, amines, glycosides, oxalates, resins, toxalbumins, minerals, and compounds causing photosensitivity. Plants may cause poisoning by (1) inducing local symptoms of mechanical or chemical irritation, (2) by absorption of active principles and systemic toxicity due to effect on one or more target organs, and (3) by allergic and hypersensitivity reactions. Actions of the more common plants causing toxicity are discussed in this chapter. Common toxic and nontoxic plants are listed in Tables 17-1 and 17-2, respectively.

Poisoning

Numerous plants contain gastrointestinal irritant agents. Among the commonest are plants of the genera *Dieffenbachia* (dumb cane) and Philodendron, which irritate the throat and gastrointestinal tract because they contain microscopic crystals of calcium oxalate in their tissue. The irritation may be severe enough to paralyze the vocal cords. These crystals occur in the *Dieffenbachias* and in all the plants belonging to the Araceae plant family. Bird of paradise and poinsettia are two other plants that produce mild gastrointestinal irritation. The irritation produced by pokeweed is so severe that it leads to hemorrhagic gastritis.

Poison oak, ivy, and sumac have a resin, urushiol, containing the allergen pentadecylcatechol that produces an allergic skin irritation. Thus, the irritation produced is not due to a direct irritant but to an allergic reaction (contact dermatitis). Poison ivy is a vine or a shrub with leaves in groups of three in which two of the leaves are directly opposed and the third leads off of the stem. Poison oak is a vine or low shrub with leaves in groups of three similar to poison ivy, but the leaves are lobed, and the underside of the leaves are lighter colored because of their fine hairs. Poison sumac is a woody shrub whose leaves consist of 7 to 13 pairs of leaflets and a single leaflet at the end of the stem.

TABLE 17-1: COMMON TOXIC PLANTS

PLANT	TOXICITY RATING*	TOXIC PART OF PLANT
Acorn (oak)	2	Tannins (toxic when uncooked)
Azalia	2	All parts
Belladonna	4	All parts
Bittersweet	4	All parts
Buckeye	4	Leaves, flowers, seeds, sprouts
Castor bean	4	Seed (if chewed)
Deadly nightshade	4	All parts
Dieffenbachia (dumb cane)	2	All parts
Elderberry	3	Roots, stems, leaves, flowers, and unripe berries
English ivy	3	Leaves, berries
Euonymus	3	Leaves, bark, and seeds
Four-o'-clock	3	Root, seed
Foxglove (digitalis)	4	Seeds, leaves
Hemlock (water)	4	All parts
Holly	3	Berries
Hyacinth	3	All parts, especially bulbs
Jequirty bean	4	Seeds
Jerusalem cherry	4	Leaves and unripe fruit
Jimsonweed	4	All parts, especially seeds and leaves
Lantana	4	Fruit, particularly unripe fruit
Larkspur	3	Seeds, young plants
Lily of the valley	4	Leaves, flowers, roots, and fruit
Mistletoe	4	Berries
Mulberries	2	Unripe berries
Philodendron	2	All parts
Poison ivy	1	Leaves
Pokeweed (poke berries)	3	Roots, stems, uncooked leaves, and berries
Rhododendron	2	All parts
Rhubarb	3	Leaves
Rubber tree	1	Milky sap
Sorrel	3	All parts
Tulip	1	Bulb
Wisteria	3	Seeds, pods
Yew	4	Berries

*TOXICITY RATINGS are as follows:
1. **Dermatitis Producing.** A rash occurring due to either a simple chemical irritation, a hypersensitive reaction, or both.
2. **Mildly Toxic.** Usually local gastrointestinal symptoms; possibly nausea and vomiting; no serious effects expected.

3. **Moderately Toxic.** Local gastrointestinal irritation, with possible systemic effects resulting from ingestion of significant amounts.
4. **Highly Toxic.** Serious systemic effects from ingestion of even small amounts.

TABLE 17-2: COMMON NONTOXIC PLANTS

Abelia	Dogwood	Pagoda plant
Absynnian sword lily	Donkey tail	Painted lady
African daisy	Dracaena palm	Painted needle
African palm	Easter lily	Palms
African violet	Emerald ripple	Passion plant
Airplane plant	Escheveria	Peacock plant
Aluminum plant	Eugenia	Peperomia
Aralia	False aralia	Petunia
Araucaria	Fiddleleaf fig	Piggyback plant
Asparagus fern	Forsythia	Prayer plant
Aspidistra (cast iron plant)	Gardenia	Purple passion
Aster	Geranium	Purple tiger
Baby's tears	Ghost plant	Pyracantha
Bachelor buttons	Giant white inch plant	Raspberries
Bamboo	Gloxinia	Rose bush
Barberries	Goldfish plant	Rose of Sharon
Bear feet	Gout weed	Rubber plant
Begonia	Grape ivy	Schefflera
Birdnest sansevieria	Hedge apple	Sedum
Bird's nest fern	Hens and chicks	Silver tree
Blackberries	Honey locust	Silver leaf
Bloodleaf	Honeysuckle	Snake plant
Boston fern	Hoya	Spider plant
Bougainvilla	Impatiens (impatience plant)	String of hearts
Bridal veil	Indian laurel	String of pearls
Buddleia (butterfly plant)	Jade plant	Swedish ivy
Calathea	Janet Craig	Ti plant
California holly	Kalanchoe	Tiger lily
California poppy	Lipstick plant	Umbrella plant
Camelia	Live forever	Velvet plant
Chinese monkey tree	Madagascar dragon	Venus fly trap
Christmas cactus	Madagascar lace plant	Violets
Coleus	Magnolia	Wandering Jew
Corn plant	Marigold	Warneckei plant
Crab apple	Mimosa	Wax plant
Creeping charlie	Mock orange	Weeping fig
Creeping jenny	Monkey plant	Weeping willow
Dahlia	Moon magic	Wild onion
Daisies	Mother-in-law tongue	Yucca
Dandelion	Mulberries (when ripe)	Zebra plant
Day lily	Norfolk island pine	

Akee is a tropical plant with a polypeptide that is responsible for the vomiting sickness indigenous to Jamaica. One unripe fruit contains a lethal dose of the poison, which is soluble in boiling water. The clinical manifestations are nausea, vomiting, and abdominal discomfort beginning 2 hours after ingestion, followed by convulsion, hypoglycemia, coma, and shock.

The castor bean and jequirty bean contain the toxalbumins ricin and abrin, respectively, which produce agglutination and hemolysis of red blood cells. After 1 to 3 days the patient develops nausea, vomiting, diarrhea, cyanosis shock, and oliguria. The latter progresses to uremia up to 12 days after ingestion.

Hemlocks are poisonous plants containing the resins coniine (poison hemlock, *Conium maculatum*) and cicutoxin (water hemlock, *Cicuta maculata*) and are among the most poisonous plants in the world. The former causes neuromuscular paralysis similar to curare paralysis, and the latter stimulates the central nervous system, causing convulsions similar to picrotoxin stimulation.

The major toxic mushrooms are *Amanita muscaria* and *Amanita phalloides*. One to 2 hours after ingestion *Amanita muscaria* produces muscarine poisoning with severe parasympathetic stimulation (salivation, lacrimation, urination, defecation, and even convulsions and pulmonary edema). *Amanita phalloides*, after a latent interval of 12 to 24 hours, produces severe nausea, bloody vomiting, and diarrhea followed by liver and renal damage accompanied by hypoglycemia, coma, and convulsions.

Several of the plants of the genera *Veratrum* (e.g., false hellebore) and *Zigadenus* (e.g., death camas) contain nitrogenous compounds that slow the heart and lower the blood pressure. Chronic use of the veratrum alkaloids to treat hypertension may lead to muscle spasm and neuropathy. Acute large doses of these alkaloids may raise the blood pressure by direct effect on the vasomotor center of the brain.

Various plants contain photosensitizing compounds (e.g., furocoumarin). The furocoumarins are useful in the treatment of vitiligo, but they are hepatotoxic.

Treatment

As stated earlier, most plants are not very toxic, but for any significant exposure, follow the general principles discussed in Chapter 2.

Some particular situations call for specific treatment. Treat the contact dermatitis of poison ivy, oak, and sumac with antipruritic and anti-inflammatory agents such as topical steroids. In severe cases administer systemic corticosteroids.

In poisonings with the castor or jequirty bean, alkalinize the urine with sodium bicarbonate to prevent precipitation of hemoglobin and its products in the kidney. In ingestion of water hemlock, treat any seizures with anticonvulsant agents. In ingestion of poison hemlock, the patient may need mechanical respiratory assistance. When *Amanita muscaria* is ingested, the patient may require atropine; and in *Amanita phalloides* ingestion, two new specific antidotes are thioctic acid and cytochrome C. When plants of the genera *Veratrum* and *Zigadenus* are ingested, atropine will block the reflexive fall in blood pressure and the bradycardia. If hypertension is present, a sympathetic blocking agent may be needed.

References — Chapter 17

J. M. Arena, "Pretty Poisonous Plants." *Vet. Hum. Toxicol.* 21:108-112, 1979.

U.S. Department of Health and Human Services, *Common Poisonous and Injurious Plants.* (Washington, DC: U.S. Government Office, 1981).

U.S. Public Health Service Publication No. 1220. *Common Poisonous Plants of New England.* (Washington, DC: U.S. Government Printing Office, 1964).

J. W. Hardin, and J. M. Arena, *Human Poisoning from Native and Cultivated Plants.* (Durham, NC: Duke University Press, 1969).

P. A. Kinamore, R. W. Jaeger, and F. J. deCastro, "Abrus and Ricinus Ingestion: Management of 3 Cases." *Clin. Toxicol.* 17:401-406, 1980.

J. M. Kingsbury, *Poisonous Plants of the United States and Canada.* (Englewood Cliffs, NJ: Prentice-Hall, 1964).

K. F. Lampe, and R. Fagerstrom, *Plant Toxicity and Dermatitis: A Manual for Physicians.* (Baltimore: Williams & Wilkins, 1968).

Poisonous Plants Around the Home, Florida Experimental Station Bulletin, 1966.

Poisonous Plants of Florida, Florida Experimental Station Bulletin, 1952.

Poisonous Plants of Georgia, Bulletin of the University of Georgia School of Veterinary Medicine, 1949.

Poisonous Plants of Pennsylvania, Pennsylvania Department of Agriculture, 1965.

The Sinister Garden. (New York: Wyeth Laboratories, 1968).

CHAPTER 18 *ANIMAL TOXINS*

Animals that contain toxin or venom are scattered throughout the different animal phyla from unicellular protozoa to complex animals. The most common animals with toxin include reptiles such as snakes and Gila monsters, insects and arachnids such as hymenoptera, spiders, and scorpions, and marine animals such as mollusks and fish.

SNAKES

Poisonous snakes are common in tropical and semitropical areas of the world, but they also live in temperate zones. Snake venoms are mostly protein, and some have enzymatic activities. The venom actions are cytotoxic, producing both local tissue damage and damage to red blood cells and organs such as the heart and kidney; neurotoxic, producing both central effects — convulsions and respiratory and cardiac depression — and peripheral neuromuscular paralysis; and coagulotoxic, producing bleeding diathesis.

The type of venom as well as the clinical picture of the patient varies with the type of snake. Snakes from the Crotalidae family such as rattlesnakes, the water moccasins (cottonmouth), and copperheads produce mostly cytotoxic changes at the site of the bite. Swelling, edema, and pain develop promptly and are followed by discoloration, ecchymosis, petechia, and hemorrhagic bullae.

Poisoning

One method of determining the severity of the bite is as follows. If the swelling is less than 12 inches in 12 hours, consider the bite grade I. If the swelling is more than 12 inches in 12 hours, the bite is Grade II. In Grade III bites, systemic symptoms of nausea, vomiting, sweating, and fainting occur, in addition to the large, rapid swelling. In Grade IV bites, cardiovascular collapse occurs, as well as all the aforementioned symptoms and swelling. Crotalidae bites are the most common in the United States, except in Florida, where coral snake bites are also common. A more useful method of grading snakebite from midwestern snakes is the following:

Minimal Envenomations

1. Manifestations remain confined to or around the bite area (local edema, pain, erythema rarely progresses beyond an inch or so within 6 hours)

2. No systemic signs and symptons

3. No laboratory changes

Moderate Envenomations

1. Manifestations extend beyond immediate bite area (severe pain, tenderness, edema 10 to 15 inches, erythema, petechiae)

2. Significant systemic signs and symptoms (vomiting, fever, weakness)

3. Moderate laboratory changes, i.e., decreased fibrinogen and platelets, and hemoconcentration

Severe Envenomations

1. Manifestations involve entire extremity or part (widespread pain, tenderness, edema 15 inches or more, ecchymosis)

2. Serious systemic signs and symptoms (vertigo, central nervous system symptoms, visual disturbances, shock, convulsions)

3. Very significant laboratory changes

Bites from snakes of the Elapidae family such as the cobras and coral snakes are characterized by rapid onset of neurotoxicity without significant local toxicity. The neurotoxicity is usually manifest by paralysis, shock, and respiratory depression beginning within an hour of the bite. Coral snakes are common in Florida. Although sea snakes are not of practical consideration here because they are not indigenous to the United States, they are of clinical interest because the bite of this snake produces significant neurotoxicity associated with myoglobinuria. Also clinically interesting are the Old World venomous snakes of the Viperidae family whose bite causes not only local cytoxic damage but also bleeding diathesis.

Treatment

Emergency measures in snake bite should include immobilization of the part and washing of the bitten area. Incision through the fang marks with mechanical suction is beneficial if done within 20 minutes of the bite; however, cross cutting unnecessarily damages structures. Applying a tourniquet and hypothermia are controversial and can cause more damage than good. Prophylaxis against tetanus and preventive and therapeutic measures against infection are always important in treating snake bite.

Specific antiserum (after the patient is tested for sensitivity) can be lifesaving but can also produce significant allergic reaction and even anaphylaxis, since snake antiserum is horse serum. Certainly antiserum is not needed in grade I Crotalidae bites, in which the major problem is local tissue damage, which may, however, include impairment of the circulation to the involved area and require dependent drainage. In severe cases surgical decompression of the local vessels may be necessary.

Of bites from pit vipers, 20 to 30 percent may be "dry," with no evenomation, requiring only local wound care and observation for 4 to 6 hours. Patient may be discharged after 6 hours if no symptoms occur.

When pharmacologic treatment is indicated, the definitive treatment is antivenin (antivenom, antivenum, antivenene, antivenine) therapy. Wyeth Polyvalent Antivenin is prepared from purified horse serum following hyperimmunization of horses to snake venom. The antivenin is made from venom of pit viper species found in the western hemisphere, which contain most of the antigens found in other pit vipers throughout the world. Thus, polyvalent antivenin is effective against all North and South American pit vipers. A dangerous complication of antivenin use is hypersensitivity (see below). A new monovalent, polyclonal F(AB) fragment antivenin is under investigation and has been reported to produce fewer allergic reactions. However, it is not yet available for general use.

Surgical treatment including excision, incision and suction, and fasciotomy are adjuncts but are not the treatment of choice. The timing and method of these procedures are controversial. When antivenin is used it is always given intravenously diluted in parenteral fluids. The package insert describes intramuscular (gluteal) administration, but it is never used in practice in the United States. For patients who demonstrate hypersensitivity or allergy to horse serum, the package insert also describes a method of "desensitization" by subcutaneous administration of diluted antivenin. This also is not recommended in the recent literature. A more current procedure in patients sensitive to horse serum is the simultanous administration of epinephrine at a rate of 1 microgram/kg/min for the first 30 minutes to 1 hour that the antivenin is given (see below).

Give the total estimated dose of antivenin as early as possible, within the first 4 to 6 hours following envonomation. For minimal envenomations (with the exception of the copperhead, whose bites should require no treatment) 3 to 5 vials may be given over 1 hour. Antivenin is not considered effective after 24 hours and may even be dangerous. However, it has been used to reverse coagulopathy occuring after 24 hours.

Children and the elderly require at least as much antivenin as adults and may need more because they have smaller extracellular volume to dilute venom, less tissue mass to slow the spread of the venom, and less protein to bind the venom.

Unlike other drugs, the dose of antivenin is based on clinical findings rather than age or weight. However, base the amount of fluid it is given in on weight or body surface area.

Sensitivity to horse serum is a serious, even life-threatening, complication. The incidence of allergic reactions is reported to be as high as 20 percent and is influenced by the amount and rate of antivenin given and the patient's age. In addition to the immediate risk of anaphylaxis, most patients receiving more than 5 vials of antivenin will develop serum sickness, usually 5 to 15 days after treatment is begun. Follow the procedure below to determine sensitivity and proceed with administration of the antivenin only when it is essential.

Determining sensitivity to horse serum
1. Test for sensitivity: 0.02 ml (one third minimum) of 1:10 horse serum from test vial, included with vial of antivenin, or make a 1:10 dilution of mixed antivenin.
2. Check site at least every 5 minutes for reaction.
3. Positive reaction is a wheal and flare with or without pruritis, pseudopodia, or systemic manifestations of allergy.

Administering antivenin if the patient tests positive on the skin test or has a history of horse serum allergy
1. Weigh the benefit of antivenin against the risk of a possibly fatal allergic reaction.
2. Preadminister Benadryl, 50 mg intravenously initially; repeat every 2 to 4 hours, not exceeding 400 mg/24 hrs.
3. Start an infusion of intravenous epinephrine and run concurrent with antivenin in an extremity opposite the bite, at a rate of 1 microgram/kg/min by I-MED or Harvard Pump. Epinephrine administration is usually necessary only for the first 30 minutes to 1 hour.

GILA MONSTER

The Gila monster is the only poisonous lizard indigenous to

the United States. Its venom produces local swelling and neurotoxicity accompanied by weakness and respiratory depression. Furthermore, the lizard's jaw muscles are so strong that even after it dies these muscles may need to be cut to remove the animal from the victim. No specific antidote is available; treatment is symptomatic only.

INSECTS

Insects are vectors of diseases such as yellow fever, plague, and Rocky Mountain spotted fever. The sting of insects of the Hymenoptera family such as bees, wasps, and hornets is also an important cause of anaphylaxis. The stinging mechanism usually consists of an acid gland containing formic acid and an alkaline gland containing convulsant factors and a histaminelike substance. The toxicity of the venom is not great and is usually responsible for local swelling and redness only. However, some persons may also be sensitized by the sting to the protein of the venom or of the insect's body. Subsequent exposure may result in life-threatening, allergic reaction such as anaphylaxis, which must be treated as any anaphylactic reaction with epinephrine and other lifesaving measures (see Chap. 2).

Furthermore, if after being stung by an insect such as a bee, wasp, or hornet, the patient develops signs of systemic or generalized allergic reactions such as urticaria, bronchospasm, and swelling of an entire extremity, hyposensitization is most likely necessary to prevent possible death.

ARACHNIDS

Included in the arachnids are spiders and scorpions. The two important spiders from the toxicologic standpoint are the black widow (*Latrodectus mactans*) and the brown recluse (*Loxosceles reclusa*).

The black widow is black and has a globular abdomen marked with an orange or red hourglass-shaped spot on the ventral surface. The venom is a neurotoxin that produces muscle spasm and difficulty in swallowing followed by an ascending paralysis accompanied by difficulty in breathing. Death is unlikely. There is a specific antiserum for treatment. Calcium gluconate administered intravenously has been recommended to relieve accompanying muscle spasm.

The brown recluse spider is a yellow to medium or dark

brown spider with a darker brown patch shaped like a violin on its dorsal cephalothorax surface. Its venom is predominantly a vasoconstrictor substance similar to norepinephrine that produces ischemic cutaneous necrosis at the site of the bite. The bite is typically painless. Pain develops during the subsequent 5 hours. Systemic signs and symptoms are rare but may include cyanosis, hemoglobinuria, fever, weakness, and even delirium. There is neither a need for antiserum nor one available. Vasodilatation with phentolamine has been tried, but there is no evidence that this drug is effective. It may have some value if it is given soon after the bite occurs and before ischemic necrosis begins. Dapsone is a drug that has shown promise in clinical trials, but requires more investigation. Systemic corticosteroids are also recommended to decrease inflammatory changes around the bite. Antibiotics may be required if infection develops.

In the United States scorpions are a problem mostly in the Southwest. The toxicity of some scorpions is greater even than that of most snakes. Fortunately, scorpions inject only a very small dose. In severe cases neurotoxicity develops promptly with feeling of a thick tongue, spasm of the throat, abdominal cramps, muscle spasm, fibrillation, and even convulsion and respiratory failure. Death is rare. Specific antiserum is available.

MARINE ANIMALS

Poisonous marine animals include the mollusks and crustaceans (shellfish) and certain fish. Marine animals are the source of three major toxins: ciguatotoxin, saxitoxin, and tetrodotoxin. Scombroid poisoning is an old term for the histaminelike substance (saurine) that produces a clinical picture similar to a sensitivity reaction with urticaria and other allergic manifestations. The histidine in fish is converted through spoilage to the histaminelike substance saurine, which then causes the urticaria and other allergic manifestations. However, true fish and seafood allergy does exist.

Ciguatotoxin is found in a number of tropical fish that are usually nonpoisonous but become poisonous during certain times of the year by feeding on marine organisms that have been contaminated by benthic blue-green algae. There is no way, except by the time of the year, to predict the presence of ciguatotoxin, and these fish should not be eaten when they are not "in season." Ciguatotoxin produces cholinesterase inhibitors that cause vomiting, muscular paralysis, and even convulsions. The treatment is symptomatic.

Puffer fish, trigger fish, and parrot fish are always poisonous. The toxin they produce, tetrodotoxin, is neurotoxic and causes severe vomiting, muscular paralysis, and convulsions. Treatment is symptomatic.

Shellfish can become poisonous by feeding on certain dino-flagellastes. Shellfish toxin, saxitoxin, is especially concentrated during the spawning season. Ingestion of saxitoxin produces symptoms similar to those seen in ciguatotoxin poisoning but more severe, causing vomiting, muscular paralysis, ataxia, weakness, and even convulsions and respiratory depression. Treatment is symptomatic.

References — Chapter 18

R. Bugrus, et al., "Clinical Observation on 3,009 Cases of Ciguatera." *Am. J. Trop. Med. Hyg.* 28:1067-1070, 1970.

B. W. Halstead, *Poisonous and Venomous Marine Animals of the World. Vol. 1. Invertebrates.* (Washington, DC: U.S. Government Printing Office, 1965).

E. J. Otten, "Antivenin Therapy in the Emergency Department." *Am. J. Emerg. Med.* 1·83-93, 1983.

J. H. Pearn, "First Aid for Snake Bite: Efficacy of Constrictive Bandage with Limb Immobilization." *Med. J. Aust.* 2:293-296, 1981.

J. H. Pearn, "Survival After Snake Bite with Prolonged Neurotoxic Envenomation." *Med. J. Aust.* 2:259-261, 1971.

Poisonous Snakes of the World. U.S. Department of the Navy, Navmed P-5099. (Washington, DC: U.S. Government Printing Office, 1968).

F. E. Russell, "Clinical Aspects of the Snake Venom Poisoning in North America." *Toxicology* 7:33-38, 1969.

N. Sadan, and B. Soroker, "Observations on the Effects of the Bite of Venomous Snakes on Children and Adults." *J. Pediatr.* 76:711-715, 1970.

H. Scholer, and M. Wuthrich, "Klinische and toxikologishe probleme der Beisse durch Giftschlangen (*Vipera aspis*)." *Schweiz. Med. Wochenschr.* 100:1761-1766, 1970.

"Symposium on Snake-Bite." *Clin. Toxicol.* 3:347-512, 1970.

G. S. Wasserman, and P. C. Anderson, "Loxoscelism and Necrotic Arachnidism." *Clin. Toxicol.* 21:451-472, 1983-1984.

G. S. Wasserman, and C. J. Siegel, "Loxoscelism (Brown Recluse Spider Bite): A Review of the Literature." *Clin. Toxicol.* 14:353-358, 1977.

J. M. Yunginger, "Advances in the Diagnosis and Treatment of Stinging Insects." *All. Pediatr.* 67:325-329, 1981.

CHAPTER 19 *FOOD POISONING AND ADDITIVES*

Food poisoning is a term applied to certain illnesses of abrupt evolution, enteric in nature, and acquired through consuming food. Included are diseases produced by bacterial growth such as staphylococcal and clostridial toxins (*Staphylococcus aureus, Clostridium botulinum*, and *Clostridium perfringens*); by microorganisms such as salmonella and streptococcus; by organic substances that may occur in natural foods such as in mushrooms, ergot, and fish, and by chemical contaminants such as heavy metals and fluorides. Some people, such as those with glucose-6-phosphate dehydrogenase (G-6-PD) deficiency, also have idiosyncratic reactions to certain foods (allergic illness). *Ptomaine* is an old-fashioned term for food poisoning. Ptomaines are ammonia-substituted compounds caused by decomposition of protein by bacterial action. Only a few food poisonings are due to ptomaine. This chapter discusses not only food poisoning but also those substances added to food to improve or preserve the original quality (e.g., color) such as sodium nicotinate and nitrate, to improve flavor (e.g., with artificial sweetener), or to increase yield (e.g., by giving diethylstilbestrol to meat-producing cattle).

FOOD POISONING

Food poisoning is an acute-onset illness following ingestion of food contaminated by bacterial toxins or organisms, by chemical substances, or by naturally occurring organic substances. A few food poisonings are idiosyncratic.

The most common bacterially produced toxins in food poisoning are those manufactured by *Staphylococcus aureus, Clostridium botulinum* (botulism), and *Clostridium perfringens. Staphylococcus* food poisoning is the most common. After eating a food contaminated with staphylococci that have been allowed to proliferate in the food and produce the exotoxin (e.g., potato salad kept at room temperature for several hours), the patient has violent nausea, vomiting, and diarrhea within 2 to 4 hours after ingestion. Heating the food kills the *Staphylococcus* organisms but usually does not destroy the toxin. The best method of control is adequate refrigeration of perishable food. Treatment is symptomatic.

Clostridium perfringens produces an illness similar to staphylococcol food poisoning, but the incubation period is usually 8 to 24 hours after ingestion of the food. Treatment is also preventive, i.e., adequate refrigeration, and symptomatic.

Clostridium botulinum produces the most severe food poisoning. After an incubation period of 12 to 36 hours after ingestion this toxin causes nausea, vomiting, and diarrhea, followed by neuromuscular paralysis at the motor end-plates, which first shows as fatigue, ptosis, and dysarthria and ends in respiratory paralysis. Prevention of botulism depends on examining canned food for abnormal taste, odor, gas, turbidity, and softening and, when possible, heating home-canned foods for 15 minutes. The toxin is heat stable. There is a specific botulinus antitoxin.

Two organisms cause food poisoning not by producing an exotoxin but by proliferating first in the contaminated food and then in the patient's gastrointestinal tract, causing infectious gastroenteritis. These two organisms include several of the *Salmonella* strains and numerous *Streptococcus*. The latter have an incubation period of approximately 4 hours; the former, a period of 8 to 24 hours. The treatment is preventive, i.e., proper sanitation and cooking of food, and symptomatic.

Chemical contamination of food may also produce acute violent gastroenteritis and has an incubation period even shorter than that of staphylococcal food poisoning. Cadmium, tin, zinc, and antimony are the most frequent culprits, but lead, arsenic, mercury, and fluoride can also cause food poisoning. Furthermore, numerous ingested chemical substances produce chronic toxicity. For example, the polynuclear hydrocarbons present in charcoal-grilled steaks have been implicated as a cause of carcinoma of the stomach, and the environmentally persistent polychlorinated biphenyls used as insulators on electrical equipment produce dermatitis, nephritis, hepatitis, progressive weakness, and coma (see Chap. 15).

Plant fungi and seafoods may also contain naturally occurring organic substances that can cause food poisoning. The most important are the mushrooms of the *Amanita* genus, which produce severe nausea and vomiting; plants such as water hemlock, rhubarb leaves, and sprouted potatoes, which produce acute gastroenteritis; the fungus *Claviceps purpurea* growing in rye meal and bread, which causes ergotism characterized by abdominal cramps, gangrenous vasoocclusion, and mental stimulation; and marine animals, which can cause severe vomiting and other manifestations (see Chap. 17).

Specific persons, such as those with G-6-PD deficiency, develop hemolysis when they eat certain foods such as fava beans. Certain persons are also allergic to specific foods. The topic of food allergy is controversial and not within the scope of this book.

FOOD ADDITIVES

Food additives are substances added to food to increase the shelf life, to maintain or improve the original condition or flavor, or to increase the yield.

Benzoic acid, widely used as a food preservative, is relatively nontoxic and tasteless. A concentration of 0.1 percent prevents bacterial growth. Large doses of benzoic acid may cause gastric irritation and a clinical picture similar to salicylate poisoning (see Chap. 6).

Both sodium nicotinate and nitrate are used to color and to preserve meat. Sodium nicotinate has been responsible for outbreaks of food poisoning characterized by cutaneous vasodilation (feeling of heat and flushing) together with a dry mouth, lip swelling, and painful extremities. Sodium nitrates have resulted in outbreaks of methemoglobenemia, which in occasional cases has been fatal.

Monosodium glutamate is responsible for the so-called "Chinese restaurant syndrome" characterized by shuddering and headache after ingestion of food containing this additive.

Artificial sweeteners are widely used to improve flavor without adding calories. The two most common have been saccharin, which is unstable in acid food and if heated leaves a bitter aftertaste, and the sodium and calcium cyclamates, which are heat and acid stable and leave no aftertaste. Cyclamates have been banned by the Food and Drug Administration (FDA) because they are in part metabolized to cyclohexylamine, a known inducer of bladder cancer. More recently saccharin has also been banned by the FDA because of its possible carcinogenic potential.

Aspartame is a synthetic chemical sweetener discovered accidentally by a G. D. Searle scientist in 1965. It exists as colorless needle-like crystals in solid form and has no bitter aftertaste. It is a "dipeptide," chemically composed of two amino acids, and is a protein in all essential respects. It has the same food value of four calories to the gram as table sugar (sucrose) but is 180 times sweeter on a weight basis, thus requiring much less per use. Its use is controversial because of its metabolism in the human body to two other chemicals, both known to exert toxic effects. Aspartame itself is not absorbed into the blood stream.

It is degraded in the gastrointestinal tract to methanol and asperyl phenylalanine. While methanol is poisonous, the amounts produced by aspartame are insignificant under normal circumstances. For example, a liter (approximately one quart) of soft drink sweetened with aspartame would contain only one third the amount of methanol found in a quart of normal fruit juice (since fruits naturally contain small amounts of methanol). The other chemical, phenyalanine, is toxic to people with a genetic deficiency called PKU (phenylketonuria). These people do not have an enzyme necessary to prevent the accumulation of phenylalanine and its breakdown products in the brain. This produces a syndrome of mental deficiency, seizures, muscular twitching, hyperactivity, brain wave abnormalities, and growth retardation. However, the amount of phenylalanine produced by a quart of soft drink sweetened with aspartame is equivalent to the amount of phenylalanine found in a single egg or one ounce of cheddar cheese. Therefore, while there is a real and definite danger for persons with PKU, and it is agreed that these patients should entirely avoid consumption of aspartame just as they do other foods, the amounts required to produce serious toxicity, even in these individuals, is enormous considering expected levels of consumption.

One last concern over aspartame is whether or not it produces brain tumors according to some early charges that the company's (G. D. Searle) animal studies were invalid. However, these studies have since been repeated by independent researchers and have apparently convinced the FDA to rule out the possibility that aspartame causes brain tumors in long term use.

To increase the efficiency of meat production, cattle were fed diethylstilbesterol. However, this practice is now banned by the FDA because of a definite association between estrogen and gynecologic cancer.

Sulfites, or "sulfiting agents," are used in a number of drug products and foods as antioxidants. Sulfites are used in many processed foods including fruit drinks, beer, wine, baked goods, and dried fruits and vegetables and in the processing of some food ingredients, including gelatin, beet sugar, corn sweeteners, and food starches. Since 1959, six sulfiting agents have been listed as Generally Recognized as Safe (GRAS) by the FDA for use in food: sulfur dioxide, sodium sulfite, sodium and potassium bisulfite, and sodium and potassium metabisulfite. As of July 9, 1986, the FDA had received hundreds of reports of adverse reactions, including 19 deaths, reportedly caused by ingestion of sulfites in foods. Although sulfites are not considered a hazard to most people, as many as one million Americans, most of them asthmatics, could suffer adverse reactions if they consume them in food. Reactions have included nausea, diarrhea, anaphylactic shock, acute asthma attacks, and loss of consciousness, which occurred soon after eating restaurant salads or other food, eating certain processed foods, and drinking wine or other beverages.

FDA has taken two major steps to protect consumers who are sensitive to sulfites in food. No longer can these preservatives be used on raw fruits and vegetables. And many more processed foods containing sulfites will have to say so on the package label.

The ban on the use of sulfites on raw fruits and vegetable, excluding potato products, became effective in 1986. This regulation is aimed primarily at restaurant salad bars and other food service outlets, including grocery stores and supermarkets that use sulfites on raw produce. The ban on sulfites in fruits and vegetables does not necessarily eliminate the preservatives from other foods often featured in salad bars. Such products as potato and shrimp salads, canned vegetables and fruits, dried fruit, pickled vegetables, pickles, pickle relish, and olives all may still contain sulfites.

The new labeling regulation became effective in January 1987 and further defines when the presence of sulfites must be declared in a finished food. Any food that contains at least 10 parts per million of sulfites must identify the sulfite in the ingredient list on the label. FDA established 10 parts per million as the label declaration because that is the lowest level at which sulfites can readily be measured.

References — Chapter 19

F. L. Byran, *Diseases Transmitted by Foods.* (Atlanta, GA: Public Health Service, Centers for Disease Control, 1971).

J. G. Davis, "Food Additives: An Introductory Paper on General Problems." In *Chemical Additives in Products.* R. W. Goodwin, ed., (Boston: Little, Brown, 1967).

I. Hiromo, "Natural Carcinogenic Products of Plant Origin." *CRC Cort. Rev. Toxicol.* 8:235-240, 1981.

C. Jelinek, "Occurence and Methods of Consideration of Chemical Contaminants in Foods." *Environ. Health Perspect.* 39:143-150, 1981.

C. W. Lecos, "Sulfites: FDA Limits Uses, Broadens Labeling." *FDA Consumer* 20:11-13, 1986.

T. Suginiya, et al., "Mutagenic Factors in Cooked Foods." *CRC Cort. Rev. Toxicol.* 6:189-195, 1979.

I. A. Wolff, and A. E. Wasserman, "Nitrates, Nitrites and Nitroamides." *Science* 177:15-19, 1972.

INDUSTRIAL AND OCCUPATIONAL POISONS

Although the next few chapters deal with industrial and occupational poisoning, the health care professional must also consider the possible part played by the nonoccupational environment when evaluating signs and symptoms. Medications, taken therapeutically or abusively, may interact with chemicals encountered in the workplace. On the other hand, a worker may engage in hobbies after work hours that involve handling toxic substances.

Regardless of whether the environment concerned is occupational or nonoccupational, the diagnoses and management of the patient must be based on (1) a meticulously taken history, (2) knowledge of the nature and severity of the exposure, (3) signs and symptoms furnishing corroborative evidence on accuracy, and (4) supporting clinical and analytic laboratory tests indicating extent of exposure.

Also included in this section is the chapter on eye contamination. Accidental splashing or squirting of substances into the eyes is probably the commonest cause of toxic eye injuries and can cause severe and irreparable injury almost immediately. Other instances of contamination produce superficial reversible damage; still others induce apparently mild injury at first that progressively worsens after a latent period. It is important to recognize these different types of toxic action because of their bearing on prognosis and treatment.

CHAPTER 20 METAL POISONING

Of the more than 100 elements, 77 are metals and 52 of the metals are of industrial or economic importance. The progress of civilization can be measured by the increasing use of metals. Furthermore, many metals such as cobalt, copper, iron, magnesium, manganese, and zinc are essential in minute quantities for life. They activate enzymes, facilitate exchange and use of oxygen, and so forth. Many metals, even the essential ones, can function as toxins. Moreover, metal poisoning is often unrecognized, is poorly treated, and produces significant mortality and morbidity. This chapter discusses the most common metals involved in poisoning in alphabetical order, not in order of importance. Iron is discussed in Chapter 13.

ANTIMONY

Antimony, which is used in metal alloys and in the manufacture of foil, batteries, ceramics, textiles, safety matches, rodenticides, and some medicinal emetics, and stibine, which is a gas released when metal containing antimony is treated with acid, are both cytotoxic. Antimony, like mercury, arsenic, and some other metals, inhibits cellular enzymes by combining with the sulfhydryl (-SH) group. Antimony also irritates mucosa and tissues; stibine specifically irritates the central nervous system and red blood cells, causing hemolysis (see Chap. 4).

The maximum allowable concentration (MAC) for antimony in air is 0.5 mg/m³; for stibine it is 0.1 ppm. The fatal ingested dose is usually above 100 mg for an average-sized adult.

Poisoning

Acute poisoning. Antimony poisoning mainly causes acute gastroenteritis, with nausea, vomiting, and diarrhea that can be bloody. Hemorrhagic hepatitis and nephritis may also occur.

Chronic poisoning. Chronic antimony poisoning causes pruritus, skin pustules, conjunctivitis, headache, weight loss, and gum bleeding.

Treatment

The emergency measures for antimony poisoning require the basic principles of emergency care (see Chap. 2). Dimercaprol (BAL) is the specific chelating agent used in antimony poisoning. In stibine-induced hemolysis, as in all hemolytic processes, alkalinize the urine.

ARSENIC

Arsenic, which is used in insecticides, herbicides, paints, wallpapers, ceramics, medicines, and glass, and arsine, which is the gas released when arsenic-containing alloys come in contact with water, are both cytotoxic. Arsenic, like antimony, inhibits cellular enzymes by combining with the sulfhydryl (-SH) group.

Arsenic causes severe irritation of the gastrointestinal tract, degeneration of the liver and spleen, and intravascular hemolysis. A blood level above 3 micrograms/100 ml is abnormal. The MAC for arsenic in food is 0.2 mg/kg of food and for the environment is 0.05 ppm.

Poisoning

Acute poisoning. Acute arsenic poisoning causes severe gastroenteritis, with burning esophageal pain, vomiting and diarrhea that are often bloody, garlic odor in the breath, and hypotension leading to shock and convulsions. If death does not occur during shock and convulsion, the patient subsequently shows hepatic and renal failure.

Chronic poisoning. Chronically, arsenic causes polyneuritis, optic neuritis, bronzing of the skin, alopecia, deformed nails (Aldrich-Mees lines), cirrhosis of the liver, vomiting, anemia, malaise, weight loss, and chronic nephritis followed by heart failure.

Treatment

Perform emergency care as described in Chapter 2. The specific antidote is dimercaprol (BAL). In severe poisoning, dialysis combined with chelation has been reported to be beneficial.

BERYLLIUM

Beryllium is used as an agent in alloys, electrical equipment, and some fluorescent lights. It inhibits certain magnesium-activated enzymes and is also very irritating to the skin and mucous membranes. The MAC in air is 0.002 mg/m^3.

Poisoning

Acute poisoning. Acute poisoning with beryllium produces pneumonitis with chest pain, bronchospasm, cyanosis, cough, and blood-tinged sputum. Cuts with objects contaminated with beryllium can cause deep, difficult-to-heal ulcerations.

Chronic poisoning. Chronic poisoning with this metal produces malaise, weight loss, chronic pulmonary granulomatosis in which chest x-ray films resemble sarcoidosis, and skin resembling chronic eczema.

Treatment

Emergency measures are those set out in Chapter 2. Bronchospasms, and sometimes secondary bacterial pneumonia, may require treatment with bronchodilators and antibiotics. Administering systemic corticosteroids may be beneficial. Calcium edetate (Ca EDTA) has been suggested as the chelating agent of choice.

CADMIUM

Cadmium is used in alloys, plating metals, and silver solders. The cadmium on plated metal cans is soluble in acid foods such as fruit juices. Cadmium is damaging to all body cells. A characteristic finding is myalgia (muscle pain). After ingestion, the predominant changes are in the gastrointestinal tract, liver, and kidney. After inhalation, the changes are mostly in the lung. The MAC in air is 0.1 mg/m^3. Ingested doses of 10 mg have produced severe intoxication in average-sized adults.

Poisoning

Acute poisoning. Acute cadmium poisoning by ingestion produces severe gastroenteritis with nausea, vomiting, and diarrhea followed by myalgia and hepatic and renal damage. When inhaled, cadmium fumes cause acute pneumonitis that can be similar to the metal fume fever caused by zinc (see Zinc).

Chronic poisoning. Chronic poisoning from cadmium leads to weight loss, dyspnea, rales, and cyanosis as well as myalgia and liver and kidney damage. Characteristically there is loss of the sense of smell and yellow staining of the teeth.

Treatment

Emergency treatment follows that described in Chapter 2. Liver and kidney failure may also need to be managed. Ca EDTA is the chelating agent of choice. Do not use BAL because the BAL-cadmium complex has been reported to be nephrotoxic.

CHROMIUM

Chromium is used in chemical synthesis steel washing, electroplating, and leather tanning and as an antirust agent. Chromium irritates and destroys all cells. The pathologic changes are more marked on the skin and in the kidney. The MAC in air is 0.1 mg/m^3 and 5 g by ingestion for an average adult.

Poisoning

Acute poisoning. Acute chromium poisoning produces abdominal pain, vomiting, hypotension, and renal failure.

Chronic poisoning. Chronic poisoning produces eczematoid dermatitis associated with slowly healing ulcers. The incidence of lung cancer is increased in persons who work with chromium.

Treatment

Emergency care is given in Chapter 2. Anti-inflammatory agents such as aluminum acetate and topical steroids may be necessary for the eczematoid dermatitis. Ca EDTA ointment has also been recommended. BAL is the systemic chelating agent of choice.

LEAD

Lead is used in alloy-type metals (brass), storage batteries, paints, solders, electric cable coverings, pottery glazes, rubber, gasoline (tetraethyl lead), and artificial pearl coloring. Lead is also present in bootleg whiskey, dust in shooting galleries, and above all in paint chips in dilapidated houses built before World War II, before titanium oxide replaced lead in indoor paints.

Lead damages all cells, but the most serious effects are in the brain and peripheral nervous system. Lead, like antimony, arsenic, and mercury, combines with the sulfhydryl (-SH) group of cell enzymes. The MAC of lead in air is 0.2 mg/m^3 and in food is 2.56 mg/kg of food. The normal dietary intake is 0.2 to 0.4 mg of lead. Children who eat several paint chips the size of a fingernail clipping (chips painted with a paint containing more than 1 percent lead) ingest a very large dose (100 mg) of lead.

A blood lead level above 400 micrograms/100 ml indicates increased lead exposure. Determinations of intermediate metabolites of hemoglobin, such as delta-amino-levulinic acid, coproporphyrin, and free erythrocyte protoporphyrin (FEP), are screening tests to determine whether lead or other toxin interferes with bone marrow function. FEP is a screening micromethod widely used to test for lead poisoning. FEP above 60 microgram/100 ml is abnormal. Growth arrest lines or lead lines observed on x-ray films of fast-growing bones of children intoxicated with lead indicate the temporary cessation of growth.

Poisoning

Acute poisoning. Acute lead poisoning produces a metallic taste and severe gastroenteritis, with abdominal pain, vomiting, and diarrhea. Subsequently, the patient may progress to coma and renal failure.

Chronic poisoning. Chronic lead poisoning by ingestion, inhalation, and skin absorption leads early to nonspecific signs and symptoms such as anorexia, listlessness, constipation, or irritability. Later the patient develops difficulty in coordination, ataxia, and loss of recently acquired skills. Finally, in severe chronic poisoning there may be renal involvement with proteinuria and glycosuria as well as signs of peripheral neuropathy such as wristdrop and footdrop and of increased intracranial pressure such as vomiting, convulsions, and coma.

Treatment

Emergency treatment is set out in Chapter 2. Furthermore, all three major chelating agents (Ca EDTA, BAL, and penicillamine, see chelating agents, Chap. 2) are used in lead intoxication individually or in combination, depending on the particular clinical situation.

MANGANESE

Manganese is used in the production of steel and dry cell batteries. Manganese mainly affects the nervous system, producing symptoms of extrapyramidal tract disease by unknown mechanisms. The MAC in air is 5 mg/m^3.

Poisoning

Acute poisoning. Acute poisoning with manganese causes lethargy associated with early signs of Parkinson's disease.

Chronic poisoning. Chronic manganese poisoning produces extrapyramidal signs and symptoms simulating Parkinson's disease.

Treatment

Emergency care follows that prescribed in Chapter 2. Both BAL and Ca EDTA have been used as the chelating agent in manganese poisoning. Moreover, antiparkinson drugs such as levodopa have been shown to be beneficial.

MERCURY

Mercury is used in manufacturing thermometers, felts, paints, explosives, lamps, electrical equipment, batteries, insecticides, fungicides, and disinfectants. Mercury, like lead and arsenic, binds the sulfhydryl (-SH) group of cellular enzymes.

The MAC in air for mercury is 0.1 mg/m^3. The fatal ingested dose of inorganic mercury salts, like mercury chloride, for adults is approximately 1 g. Ingestion of metallic mercury, such as that in thermometers, is not toxic because it is not absorbed well from the gastrointestinal tract unless an obstruction or inflammatory disease is present. The toxicity of organic mercury compounds varies with the specific compound. For example, the toxicity of mercurial diuretics such as Mercuhydrin (meralluride) is similar to that of mercury chloride, but the toxicity of volatile diethyl and demethyl mercury compounds is ten times greater, especially in the central nervous system. Phenyl mercury compounds are similar in toxicity to mercury chloride. They are less corrosive but more volatile and therefore allow for easy intoxication by inhalation.

Methyl mercury from agricultural fungicides that contaminate lakes and subsequently fish present special problems. Toxicity with methyl mercury is insidious, with predominant effects on the central nervous system, and since the compound is bound to hemoglobin in red cells, toxicity persists for a long time. The problems of methyl mercury compounds were unrecognized until the 1960s, when the Japanese reported an epidemic of poisoning from this compound on the island of Kyushu around Minamata Bay.

Poisoning

Acute poisoning. Inhalation of volatile mercury compounds causes pneumonitis, salivation, and metallic taste. Acute ingestion of mercury compounds causes metallic taste, thirst, salivation, and corrosive gastroenteritis associated with nausea, vomiting, and bloody diarrhea. These symptoms are followed by uremia during the next few weeks. Acute mercury poisoning may also cause fatal convulsions. Methyl mercury compounds, as previously stated, have a predilection for the central nervous system, causing ataxia, tremors, and convulsions.

Chronic poisoning. Chronic mercury poisoning causes dermatitis, bone marrow depression, liver damage, and renal failure. In children, repeated administration of mercury compounds such as calomel (a cathartic) has been associated with erythema and polyneuropathy together with pink, painful extremities (acrodynia). Chronic ingestion of methyl mercury compounds, as in acute methyl mercury poisoning, also causes ataxia, tremors, and convulsions. Chronic inhalation of mercury compounds causes mercurialism, with tremors, salivation, stomatitis, loosening of teeth, and mental deterioration.

Treatment

In mercury poisoning, as in poisoning from many other metals, preventive and emergency measures are always important (see

Chap. 2). The best chelating agent for mercury intoxication is peni-cillamine. BAL has also been used successfully.

NICKEL

Nickel and its salt cause hypersensitization and irritations of the skin. Nickel carbonyl is a colorless liquid formed by passing carbon monoxide over finely divided metallic nickel. Nickel carbonyl is a by-product of nickel refining and of the manufacture of plastics. This finely divided nickel causes irritation and necrosis of the lungs and brain.

Poisoning

Acute poisoning. Acute exposure to nickel may cause hypersensitization and irritation of the skin accompanied by weeping papulovesicular lesions. Inhalation of nickel carbonyl causes cough, dizziness, headaches, cyanosis, fever, and even death from respiratory failure.

Chronic poisoning. Chronic exposure to nickel increases the incidence of lung cancer. Dermatitis is also a problem in persons who work with nickel.

Treatment

Emergency care as well as preventive measures are always important in nickel poisoning therapy (see Chap. 2). Oxygen may be needed in cyanosis due to nickel carbonyl. BAL has been used as the chelating agent, but a newer chelating agent — diethyldithiocarbamate — seems to give better results.

PHOSPHORUS

Phosphorus exists as either red phosphorus, which is non-absorbable and nontoxic, or yellow phosphorus, which is fat-soluble, absorbable, and highly toxic. Matches contain either red phosphorus or phosphorus sesquisulfide. Both are nonabsorbable and nontoxic. Yellow phosphorus is used in rodenticides, insecticides, fireworks, and fertilizers. When water and acids are poured on metals containing phosphorus, a toxic gas — phosphine — may be liberated.

Phosphorus destroys tissues and disturbs cellular carbohydrate, fat, and protein metabolism; causes liver and kidney deterioration; and erodes the gastrointestinal tract, causing hemorrhage.

The MAC of yellow phosphorus in the air is 0.1 mg/m³; for phosphines it is 0.3 ppm. The fatal oral dose of yellow phosphorus for adults is 50 mg.

Poisoning

Acute poisoning. Acute yellow phosphorus ingestion causes corrosive gastroenteritis with nausea, vomiting, and diarrhea, garlic odor of breath, and death from coma and hypotension. Renal and hepatic failure may also occur. Yellow phosphorus on the skin not only irritates but may also ignite. Inhalation of phosphine may cause hypotension, dyspnea, pulmonary edema, convulsions, and coma.

Chronic poisoning. Chronic yellow phosphorus poisoning causes toothache, necrosis of the mandible, weakness, weight loss, and anemia. Renal and liver failure may also occur.

Treatment

There is no specific chelating agent for phosphorus poisoning. Preventive and emergency measures are crucial (see Chap. 2). Symptomatic care is essential, that is, treating the pulmonary edema, administering calcium gluconate if there is hypocalcemia, treating the hepatic and renal failure, and so forth. Surgical excision of a necrosed jaw may also be required.

ZINC

Galvanized zinc cans and utensils used to prepare or store acid foods may dissolve zinc when they come in contact with those foods. Zinc fumes are produced in welding, metal cutting, and smelting zinc alloys and galvanized iron, and zinc chloride is used in smoke generators. Zinc irritates tissues; when inhaled, zinc fumes are responsible for metal fume fever. The MAC for zinc fumes in air is 15 ppm.

Poisoning

Acute poisoning. Acute inhalation of zinc fumes leads to metal fume fever, with fever, vomiting, myalgia, and pneumonitis. Muscular ache is always present in acute zinc toxicity. Pulmonary findings may range from pneumonitis to pulmonary edema associated with cyanosis and dyspnea. Toxic ingestion of zinc produces severe vomiting and diarrhea.

Chronic poisoning. To date no chronic poisoning syndrome from zinc has been described. A syndrome of hypogonadism, anemia, and hepatosplenomegaly has been described in Iranian men secondary to chronic zinc deficiency.

Treatment

Preventive and emergency measures are crucial (see Chap. 2). There is no chelating agent for zinc. Corticosteroids are recommended to treat zinc-induced pulmonary irritation.

References — Chapter 20

M. Barborik, and J. Dusek, "Cardiomyopathy Accompanying Industrial Cobalt Exposure." *Br. Heart J.* 34:113-116, 1971.

R. T. Barton, "Nickel Carcinogens of the Respiratory Tract." *J. Otolaryngol.* 6:412-415, 1977.

R. F. Carter, "Acute Selenium Poisoning." *Med. J. Aust.* 1:525-528, 1966.

S. V. Chandra, "Histological and Histochemical Changes in Experimental Manganese Encephalopathy in Rabbits." *Arch. Toxicol.* 29:29-38, 1972.

J. S. Felton, et al., "Heavy Metal Poisoning: Mercury and Lead." *Ann Intern. Med.* 76:779-792, 1972.

D. G. Freiman, and H. L. Hardy, "Beryllium Disease: The Relation of Pulmonary Pathology to Clinical Course and Prognosis Based on a Study of 130 Cases from the U. S. Beryllium Case Registry." *Hum. Pathol.* 1:25-44, 1970.

R. A. Goyer, "Lead Toxicity: A Problem in Environmental Pathology." *Am J. Pathol.* 64:167-182, 1971.

V. F. Guiness, "Lead Poisoning." *Am. J. Med.* 52:283-288, " 1972.

M. M. Joselow, D. B. Louria, and A. M. Browder, "Mercurialism: Environmental and Occupational Aspects." Ann. Intern. Med. 76:119-130, 1972.

M. E. Markovitz, and J. F. Rosen, "Assessment of Lead Stores in Children: Validation of the 8-hour CaEDTA Provocative Test." *J. Pediatr.* 104:337-341, 1984.

E. A. Mastromatteo, "Nickel: A Review of its Occupational " Health Aspects." *J. Occup. Med.* 9:127-136, 1967.

E. A. Natelson, B. J. Blumenthal, and H. L. Fred, "Acute Mercury Vapor Poisoning in the Home." *Chest* 59:677-678, 1971.

P. E. Pierce, et al., "Alkyl Mercury Poisoning in Humans." *J.A.M.A.* 220:1439-1442, 1972.

S. Pionelli, et al., "The FEP (Free Erythroctye Porphyrin) Test: A Screening Micromethod for Lead Poisoning." *Pediatrics* 12:254-259, 1973.

"Polymer-Fume Fever." *Lancet* 2:27-28, 1972.

J. St. Petery, et al., "Arsenic Poisoning in Childhood." *Clin. Toxicol.* 3:519-526, 1970.

L. T. Smyth, et al., "Clinical Manganism and Exposure to Manganese in the Production and Processing of Ferromanganese Alloy." *J. Occup. Med.* 15:101-109, 1973.

J. M. Wisniewski-Knypl, J. Jablonska, and A. Mystak, "Binding of Cadmium on Metallothionein in Man: An Analysis of a Fatal Poisoning by Cadmium Iodide." *Arch. Toxicol.* 28:46-55, 1972.

CHAPTER 21 *ATMOSPHERIC POLLUTANTS*

Air pollutants, like metal irritants, are to a great extent the result of progress. Atmospheric pollutants are substances that either are not normally present in the air, or, if present, their natural concentration is increased by human activities. The most important air pollutants are products of photochemistry such as ozone, peroxyacetyl nitrate, and aldehydes; of carbon and its oxides such as sulfur dioxide; of nitrogen and its oxides such as nitrogen dioxide; of hydrocarbons including both aliphatics (olefins) and aromatics (polycyclic ring compounds); of dusts of particulate matter such as silica and coal; and of gases, many of which are members of the above-mentioned categories.

PRODUCTS OF PHOTOCHEMISTRY

Ozone, which is an allotropic form of oxygen, peroxyacetyl nitrate (PAN), and aldehydes such as formaldehyde are all products of photochemical reaction in the atmosphere. Aliphatic hydrocarbon pollutants (olefins) and the oxides of nitrogen also enter photochemical reactions and are discussed later.

Ozone (O_3) does occur naturally in the atmosphere, but its concentration is increased by photochemical reaction in a polluted atmosphere. Ozone is the major atmospheric oxident, and it not only irritates the eyes and respiratory tract but is also responsible for cracking of rubber. It has an effect on living tissues similar to ionizing radiation. A community standard of 0.1 ppm has been set in some places. Odor threshold is at 0.05 ppm; a level above 0.1 ppm irritates the eyes of a significant number of people.

PAN and aldehydes such as formaldehyde are also products of photochemical reaction in the atmosphere. They are tissue irritants and are also responsible for disintegration of nylon clothing and marble buildings. Formaldehyde not only irritates but also stops the action of the respiratory cilia at concentrations above 0.5 ppm. Its odor can be detected at 0.05 ppm.

CARBON AND ITS OXIDES

Carbon monoxide, carbon dioxide, and soot (chains of fine carbon particles clustered together) are the most important products of carbon and its oxides present in the atmosphere. The major source of pollutants in this category is the automobile.

Carbon monoxide causes carboxyhemoglobin. Exposure to 500 ppm causes 20 percent carboxyhemoglobin in less than 1 hour. When the concentration of carboxyhemoglobin is 4 percent, there is impairment of visual contrast and interference in some psychological tests; at 20 percent the person has a headache, and at 40 percent confusion, irritability, chest pain, and fainting occur, leading to respiratory failure and death. Typically, the patient shows the cherry-red color of carboxyhemoglobin. The treatment includes breathing 100 percent oxygen and treatment of the cerebral edema. Transfusion with washed red blood cells is beneficial in severe intoxication.

Carbon monoxide is found in fairly high concentrations in urban areas. A practical rule to determine the safety of exposure is to multiply hours of exposure by parts per 10,000 of carbon monoxide concentration. If the result is 3 or less, there will be no detectable effect. Industrially, the MAC is 50 ppm, and in communities the standard maximum concentration is 20 ppm.

Carbon dioxide is not usually considered a pollutant. High concentrations as in crevices of caves can produce medullary stimulation, followed by convulsion and central nervous system depression. Carbon dioxide collects in crevices because, unlike carbon monoxide, which weighs less than air, it weighs more than air. Carbon dioxide in the presence of atmospheric moisture is converted to carbonic acid, which corrodes metals. Carbon dioxide in the atmosphere has been also implicated in slowly warming the earth.

SULFUR AND ITS OXIDES

Sulfur is present as an impurity in coal and fuel oil and thus enters the atmosphere following their combustion. The major sulfur compounds in the atmosphere are sulfur dioxide, sulfur trioxide, and sulfurous and sulfuric acids. Sulfur dioxide is the most important. It irritates tissues of the eyes and lungs and also decreases visibility by forming particulates with organic compounds and nitrogen oxides.

In communities the standard maximum concentration is 0.1 ppm. Eye irritation occurs at 10 ppm but can be recognized at 0.3 ppm, and increased resistance to breathing occurs at 1.6 ppm.

NITROGEN AND ITS OXIDES

Nitrogen is not irritating and accounts for 78 percent of the atmospheric gas, but its oxides are very irritating to the respiratory tract. Nitrogen oxides come to the atmosphere from combustion of nitrogen containing substances such as coal and fuel oil and from putrefaction of organic matter such as plant material in a silo. Cigarette smoke contains as much as 200 to 600 ppm of nitrogen oxides and pipe smoke even larger amounts. The most important oxides of nitrogen in the atmosphere are nitric oxide, nitrogen dioxide and trioxide, and nitric acid.

Nitric oxide enters into photochemical reaction with ultraviolet light and ozone and is converted to nitrogen dioxide, which is not only irritating, causing bronchiolitis fibrosa cystica (silo lung disease), but also gives smog its yellow-brown color. The MAC industrially for nitrogen dioxide is 5 ppm. In communities the standard maximum concentration is 0.25 ppm. The taste and odor thresholds are 1 ppm, and chest discomfort occurs at 15 ppm.

HYDROCARBONS

Numerous hydrocarbons pollute the air and can be divided chemically into aliphatic and aromatic compounds. Aliphatic hydrocarbons, like the olefins, enter into photochemical reaction with ozone and oxides of nitrogen. The aromatic compounds such as benzo(a)pyrene are considered carbinogenic. The main source of hydrocarbon in the atmosphere is the automobile. In communities, standard maximum concentrations of 2 ppm 90 percent of the time and 5 ppm 20 percent of the time are considered acceptable.

Chlorofluorocarbons (e.g., Freon) are nonflammable gases used as refrigerants and propellants in spray cans. Inhalation (sniffing) of high concentrations induces drowsiness, confusion, respiratory tract irritation, and epinephrine-sensitive cardiac arrhythmias. Death may occur. Chlorofluorocarbon is also implicated in destruction of the atmospheric ozone layer and the warming or cooking of the earth. For this reason, the chlorofluorocarbons have been banned from use in consumer products in the United States.

DUSTS

Dust particles or particulate matter is another category of

pollutants that must be considered. Dusts are solid particles usually ranging from 0.5 to 10 micrograms. Particles less than 5 micrograms are the most significant in regard to effect on the lower respiratory tract. Dust particles can be measured in ton per square mile or in micrograms/m^3. The most important dust particles in the air are the dusts of silica and of coal. Dusts come from many other sources such as cotton and bagasse. All the diseases caused by dust particles are classified as pneumoconioses.

Silica dust and asbestos, which is fibrous magnesium silicate (chrysotile), cause a progressive obliterative pulmonary disease. These patients not only develop pulmonary fibrosis and cor pulmonale but also have an increased incidence of progressive tuberculosis and malignant tumors. Talc is similar in composition to asbestos; that is, it is also magnesium silicate. Talc produces an illness (talcosis) similar to asbestos. Asbestos workers have an increased incidence not only of bronchogenic carcinoma but also of pleural and peritoneal mesotheliomas.

Coal workers also develop a slowly progressive fatal pulmonary disease (black lung) that terminates in pulmonary fibrosis and emphysema. Aluminum (bauxite) furnace workers also develop a progressive pulmonary fibrosis. Fumes of an aluminum furnace are also rich in silica (Shaver's disease).

The other pneumoconioses are nonprogressive pulmonary diseases that disappear when exposure is terminated. These are the diseases of cotton workers (byssinosis), of sugarcane workers (bagassosis), of farmers (farmer's lung), and so forth. Byssinosis causes bronchitis but is usually nonprogressive unless the exposure continues, and it then may lead to emphysema. Bagassosis causes pneumonitis, which is probably a hypersensitivity reaction. Farmer's lung is most likely a hypersensitivity reaction to two fungi, *Thermopolyspora polyspora* and *Micromonospora vulgaris*.

GASES

Some inhaled gases irritate the respiratory tract and sometimes even cause fatalities; others are absorbed through the alveolar membranes and cause systemic effects of different severity.

The major respiratory irritant gases are oxides of nitrogen such as nitrogen dioxide (see nitrogen and its oxides); chlorine, which is frequently generated in homes by mixing bleach (sodium hypochlorite) and an acid bowl cleaner; methyl bromide, which is used as a fumigant (see Chap. 12); ozone (see products of photochemistry); phosgene, which is generated from high-temperature decomposition of chlorinated hydrocarbons; ammonia (see Chap. 14); sulfur (sulfur and its oxides); and smoke from fires. Pulmonary edema is the usual result of lung irritation. Systemic corticosteroids have been suggested to be beneficial in patients with severe pulmonary irritation caused by significant inhalation of firesmoke and other gases.

Polymer fume fever is a disease characterized by cyanosis, dyspnea, myalgia, chest pain, and pulmonary edema, which occur after inhalation of toxic fumes emitted by polytetrafluoroethylene (Teflon) heated at high temperatures (over 506C).

Other gases cause their damage by systemic toxicity after absorption. Hydrogen cyanide and carbon monoxide are asphyxiants; that is, they induce tissue anoxia. Hydrogen cyanide stops cellular breathing by combining with the ferric iron of the cytochrome oxidase enzymes of cells, and carbon monoxide combines with hemoglobin to form carboxyhemoglobin. Other nonasphyxiating gases also cause systemic toxicity after absorption (e.g., the chlorofluorocarbons).

References — Chapter 21

S. U. Dawson, "Health Effects of Inhalation of Ambient Correlation of Nitrogen Dioxide." *Am Rev. Respir. Dis.* 120:281-286, 1979.

I. T. T. Higgins, "Effects of Sulfur Oxides and Particulates on Health." *Arch. Envir. Health* 22:584-590, 1971.

D. B. Menzel, "Toxicity of Ozone, Oxygen, and Radiation." *Ann. Rev. Pharmacol.* 10:379-394, 1970.

J. G. Terrill, Jr., E. D. Harward, and I. P. Leggett, Jr. "Environmental Aspects of Nuclear and Conventional Power Plants." *Indust. Med. Surg.* 36:412-419, 1967.

H. K. Ury, and A. C. Hexter, "Relating Photochemical Pollution to Human Physiologic Reactions Under Controlled Conditions." *Arch. Environ. Health* 18:473-480, 1969.

CHAPTER **22** *EYE CONTAMINATION*

Eye contamination from household cleaning products, industrial chemicals, and parenteral drugs (splashed into the eye during reconstitution and preparation) causes a significant number of calls to poison control centers each year.

Following a chemical splash or injury to the eye, time is of the essence. Use tap water or the first innocuous watery solution at hand to rinse and dilute the offending substance. Except for the most incidental exposures, evaluate chemical eye injuries in an emergency facility because other factors, such as mechanical injury, can contribute to corneal impairment following an accident. In the emergency room, the conjunctival sac can be continuously irrigated with sterile intravenous fluids (such as normal saline) after a topical anesthetic is administered. In chemical burns of the eye it has been suggested that cooler liquids at the beginning may help reduce the heat of some chemical reactions, but this has not been experimentally confirmed.

Since many substances do not bind chemically with tissues and are readily eliminated by irrigation, a prompt brief irrigation of several minutes should be adequate; in fact, prolonged, unnecessary irrigation may cause mechanical injury.

Prolonged irrigation is, however, strongly recommended immediately after initial contamination of the eye with alkalies, since then the pH of the conjunctival sac may take some time to return to the normal range. Test the conjunctival sac with wide-range pH test paper every 5 to 10 minutes in the course of irrigation to measure the rate at which the pH is returning to a tolerable value such as 8 or 8.5. Do not expect a pH of 7. In acid burns the pH of the conjunctival sac returns to normal range during irrigation in fewer minutes than in alkali burns. As far as is known, nothing is gained by continued irrigation after the pH has definitely returned to normal. Extended irrigation is also recommended for other chemically reactive substances or those with an oily or viscous base (e.g., hydrocarbons). When the substance is unknown, do a cautious, gentle irrigation longer than may actually be necessary rather than irrigating inadequately.

When there is a possibility of contamination with solid particles, search the conjunctival sac, completely everting the lids and removing these particles mechanically as quickly as possible, continuing irrigation concomitantly. Sweeping the fornices with a swab dabbed with a small amount of sterile ophthalmic antibiotic ointment is useful in removing particulate matter. A local anesthetic makes this procedure easier and more comfortable for the patient.

Fluorescein may be used to uncover epithelial damage on the cornea or the conjunctiva. Remember, though, that tests with fluorescein cannot be depended on to rule out injury in all cases, since symptoms of damage can be latent, sometimes for several hours after exposure. Latent periods of this sort are most commonly encountered after exposure to gases, vapors, and fumes but can also occur after contact with certain liquids and solids (e.g., ethylene oxide, hydrogen sulfides, or sodium hypochlorite-ammonia mixtures). The slit-lamp microscope and ophthalmoscope can be relied on for more detailed information in all cases of eye contamination.

Although neutralizing chemical contaminants with various reagents has been proposed, and despite its theoretical advantage, this type of neutralization has seldom been shown to provide a significant improvement over immediate irrigation with water or saline (which is usually much more readily available for first-aid treatment). There are a few instances in which specific antidotes are advantageous.

In addition to the standard treatment precautions that have already been discussed in the beginning of the chapter, the following procedures are usually the standard protocol for eye injury management:

1. Anesthesia with a suitable sterile ophthalmic eye drop.
2. Irrigation with at least 2 liters of sterile saline while the eye is held open with retractors.
3. Atropine dilatation of the eye.
4. Fluorescein staining of the cornea.
5. Therapeutic use of antibiotics.
6. Standard application of pressure patch.
7. Follow-up care as needed.

The investigational use of drugs such as l-cysteine or N-acetylcysteine to inhibit the formation of collagenase during recovery of the cornea has been attempted. Healing must occur in the first 2 weeks after injury to prevent complications due to the production of collagenase.

The following chemicals are those frequently involved in eye accidents.

ACETONE

Acetone is a volatile, highly flammable liquid with a characteristic sweetish odor. It is miscible with water, alcohol, some organic solvents, and most oils. Acetone is used in chemical manufacturing, paints, varnish solvents, cleaning fluids, and nail polish removers.

Exposure to vapor concentrations of 500 ppm produces a burning sensation in the eye but not tissue damage. Exposure to higher concentrations can cause corneal, epithelial, and conjunctival injury. A splash of a drop of liquid acetone in the human eye commonly causes an immediate stinging sensation, but if it is washed out promptly, it injures only the epithelium. This is commonly characterized by the presence of microscopic gray dots and foreign body sensation. Usually healing is complete within a day or two. Testing by application of a single drop to rabbit eyes caused reversible injury. Several drops squirted on the eyes of anesthetized rabbits and washed out 2 minutes later with water caused temporary edema and irregularity of the corneal epithelium and grayness of the stroma, but the eyes recovered completely in 2 to 5 days.

ACIDS

Sulfuric acid (oil of vitriol, battery acid) in a pure state is an odorless, colorless, oily liquid. Slight impurities produce a yellow or brown color with an unpleasant odor. Commercial preparations contain 93 to 98 percent H_2SO_4 in water. The acid is also miscible in alcohol. Dissolving sulfuric acid in either solution will generate much heat. By far the most widely used industrial chemical, sulfuric acid is used in producing fertilizers, chemicals, petroleum, iron, steel, explosives, film, and fabric, and as a common laboratory reagent.

Concentrated sulfuric acid in contact with the eye or skin appears to attack tissues chemically in a more destructive manner than is explainable by its hydrogen ion concentration. When diluted, the caustic properties become more like those of simpler acids such as hydrochloric. Fine sprays of sulfuric acid in the air cause acute stinging and burning of the eyes, but rapid dilution of tears may prevent significant injury. A 1 percent solution in water produced no permanent damage in experiments on rabbits' eyes, and transient splashes attained complete recovery within 48 hours. Severe sulfuric acid eye burns have produced glaucoma, cataracts, and dissolution of the anterior segment of the globe. The extent of the injury depends greatly on the speed with which irrigation is started.

Hydrochloric acid is hydrogen chloride in aqueous solution. It is a colorless or slightly yellow foaming, pungent liquid. The commercial reagent grade concentrated hydrochloric acid contains close to 38 percent hydrogen chloride. Technical muriatic acid is usually 32 percent, and

diluted hydrochloric acid is 10 percent. It is used in chemical manufacturing, general cleaning, industrial acidizing, and food processing.

The gas that escapes from aqueous hydrochloric acid solution is so immediately irritating to the eyes and respiratory passages that
human beings have rarely been submitted to damaging concentrations.
When a drop is splashed in the eye and immediately washed out with
water, one can observe white coagulation of the cornea and conjunctival
epithelium, but no significant damage to the corneal stroma or deeper
parts of the eye. Usually the injured epithelium comes loose in a day or
two and is replaced by new tissue. Severe cases have produced stromal
edema, opacities of the lens, and damage that results in loss of the eye.

ALKALINE CORROSIVES

Any solution above a pH of 7 containing an excess of
hydroxyl ions can be considered an alkali. Many organic amines dissociate
sufficiently to be treated as alkaline in cases of eye contact. Hair straight-
eners, although referred to as neutralizers, cause alkali burns. Phosphate-
free detergents are usually more alkaline than other detergents because
alkaline "builders" are added and can be evaluated and treated as potentially corrosive alkalies. The injuriousness of the alkali to the eye increases
greatly when the solution reaches a pH between 11 and 12, probably most
steeply at a pH of 11.5. The variation in burns between lime, lye, and
ammonia is due primarily to the differences in rate of penetration even at
an equal pH. Animal experiments suggest that the cornea with epithelium
present is penetrated from slowest to fastest in the following order:
calcium hydroxide, tetraethylammonium hydroxide, barium hydroxide,
strontium hydroxide, lithium hydroxide, potassium hydroxide, sodium
hydroxide, ammonium hydroxide.

In the acute stage there is sloughing of corneal epithelium,
necrosis of cells of the corneal stroma and endothelium, loss of corneal
mucoid, edema of the corneal stroma and the ciliary processes, ischemic
necrosis and edema of the conjunctiva and limbal region of the sclera, and
infiltration of inflammatory cells into the cornea and iris. There is a strong
tendency for corneal infiltration to develop 1 to 3 weeks after injury. Poor
results are particularly likely to result from destruction of the corneal
endothelium with resulting corneal edema, from secondary infection with
infiltration and ulceration, and from iritis and secondary glaucoma. Complications may include vascularization and scarring of the cornea, permanent opacity, retinal damage, perforation, and adhesion between the

eyelid and eyeball. If the injury has not been excessively severe, recovery will bring decreased edema, regeneration of the epithelium, clearing of corneal opacification, regeneration of endothelium, and disappearance of iritis.

BENZENE

Benzene is a volatile aromatic liquid. Generally it is not present in household products; however, it is widely used as an industrial solvent, as an additive in motor fuels, and in chemical synthetics. It is also known as benzol, phenyl hydride, coal naphtha, and phene benzol. Benzine is a different product entirely.

Droplet contamination of the eye by benzene causes a moderate burning sensation but only slight transient injury to the epithelium, from which the eye recovers rapidly. Animal data have linked high concentration of benzene vapors to cataracts. Case histories of both an acute and a chronic exposure to vapors of this aromatic hydrocarbon have suggested a "reasonably close" association between benzene poisoning and optic neuritis.

CAYENNE PEPPER OR CAPSICUM OLEORESIN

The fine powder of the dried fruit capsicum is a pungent irritant to mucous membranes and has been used therapeutically for that property in external medications. It is found primarily as a spice packaged in shaker containers.

Applying red pepper to the eye in animal experiments caused observable pain and involuntary spasm of the eye muscle. An unusual vascular response accompanied this: blood vessels in the conjunctiva and lids became abnormally permeable to dye injected intravenously. Whether this vascular change takes place in human beings is not known.

CYANOACRYLATE

Cyanoacrylic acid methyl ester is an adhesive usually available in small tubes in products such as Super Glue, Super Bonder, and Borden Ad/Here. Mucous membranes, either wet or dry, rapidly adhere to one another on exposure; there are no known solvents that reverse the polymerization process responsible for the adhesion.

Experiments designed to test this product for use in oph-thalmologic procedures found it created haze in the cornea and inflammation but generally without significant permanent damage. Tests in animals showed that the adhesive rapidly seals eyelids together, and after manual separation 24 hours after exposure, conjunctival sacs were filled with polymer and tissue exudate with significant local corneal irritation. The corneas stained with fluorescein in all animal eyes were normal within 14 days without any further treatment. Information supplied by the manufacturer indicated that when introduced into the eyes, the cyanoacrylate will attach itself to the eye protein and will disassociate from it without active medical intervention. Periods of weeping and double vision have been experienced during the time the eye is trying to clear the polymer. According to this same source, dissociation will normally occur within hours, even with gross contamination.

DETERGENTS, ANIONIC AND NONIONIC

Detergents (surfactants) are compounds having hydrophilic properties at one end of the molecule to promote water solubility and lipophilic properties at the other end to provide affinity for oils and greases. Although of varying chemical structures, they generally lower the surface tension of the water. Besides being used for cleaning, washing, and scouring, surfactants can also be found in cosmetics and antiseptics. Anionic surfactants are usually sodium salts or occasionally triethanolamine salts of alkyl sulfates or of aromatic sulfates. Many common household soaps and shampoos fall in this category. Nonionic surfactants are ester and ether combinations of fatty acids or fatty alcohols. Many surfactants are known to cause injury in contact with the eye. The anionic ones cause lysis of cells. Anionic detergents tested in rabbit eyes at 0.5 to 1 percent concentration typically caused immediate discomfort, hyperemia of the conjunctiva, edema of the corneal epithelium with punctuate stainability by fluorescein with no opacity, and prompt healing in a day or two. There is some experimental evidence at 3 percent concentrations to suggest these substances do not loosen the corneal epithelium from the stroma but gradually transform the epithelium into a slimy mass from surface to basal level. Certain of the nonionic detergents are found to have a local anesthetic action on the cornea and may damage the epithelium. Nonionic detergents in concentration usually present in household products are unlikely to produce anything more than transient irritation of the eye. A typical application of a nonionic surfactant is in vaginal contraceptive foams.

Soaps commonly produce a stinging pain and tears that cleanse the eye, with no lasting or significant injury. Phisohex has caused severe corneal edema and endothelium injury in a couple of patients, both of whom recovered in several weeks. Damage appeared to be related to the detergent rather than the hexachlorophene. In shampoo, manufacturers generally try to include ingredients that are less irritating to the eye. The sodium lauryl sulfate (an anionic detergent) in shampoo formulas is thought to be the commonest cause of eye irritation. The trend in recent years has been to reduce the pH of shampoos into the mildly acid range. This causes less swelling of the hair shaft during shampooing and makes for quicker drying, which is desirable to the consumer.

DETERGENTS, CATIONIC

As discussed earlier, detergents (surfactants) are compounds having hydrophilic properties at one end of the molecule to promote water solubility and lipophilic properties at the other end to provide affinity for oils and greases. Cationic detergents are generally quaternary ammonium derivatives, sometimes containing an organic ring.

Many surfactants are known to cause injury in contact with the eye. The cationic type precipitate protein. Testing on rabbit eyes has indicated a general but not inviolable rule that cationic detergents are the most damaging, followed by anionic and nonionic. Report of inflammation and degeneration of the iris and chorioretinitis has been made when an unknown concentration of alkenyl dimethylethyl ammonium bromide was injected into the eye of a rabbit.

Treat cationic detergents in the eye as alkaline corrosive exposures. High concentrations of cationic detergents are not generally found in the home but are usually employed in the industrial or hospital settings. These products may contain high percentages of quaternary ammonium compounds. The eyes are much more sensitive to concentrations that might otherwise be tolerated by mucous membranes or skin. Therefore, an exposure to any concentration should be followed by an ophthalmologist.

ETHYL ALCOHOL

Ethyl alcohol is a colorless liquid of pleasant odor and burning taste, moderately volatile, boiling at 78.5C. Ethyl alcohol is used in large quantities as a solvent and an antiseptic and in the manufacture of pharmaceuticals, perfumes, and cosmetics. Ethyl alcohol is also available commercially as denatured alcohol, containing various toxic substances to render it unfit for use as a beverage; the most common denaturants are methyl alcohol, camphor, acetaldol, methyl isobutyl, ketone, gasoline, kerosene, isopropyl alcohol, terpineol, benzene, castor oil, acetone, nicotine, dyes, ether, pyridine bases, and diethyl phthalate.

Splash contact of ethyl alcohol with the eye causes immediate burning and stinging sensation, with reflex closure of the lids and tearing. Splashes of distilled alcoholic beverages such as whiskey, brandy, gin, and vodka, containing 45 to 50 percent alcohol, cause transitory superficial injury, hyperemia, and discomfort. Ethyl alcohol concentrations of 70 to 90 percent, such as employed in antiseptics, astringents, lotions, colognes, and perfumes, injure the corneal epithelium and cause hyperemia of the conjunctiva. A foreign-body type of discomfort may be experienced for a day or two, but usually healing is spontaneous and complete. One instance of opacification of the cornea has been reported, but this is quite exceptional. Also an uncommonly severe reaction with corneal erosion, stromal edema, and slow recovery has been reported from a squirt of a shaving lotion that contained 50 percent alcohol plus 0.1 percent lactic acid, perfumes, ethereal oils, and glycerin.

Vapors of alcohol at sufficiently high concentrations may cause prompt stinging and watering of the eyes, but there appear to be no reports of eye injury from industrial exposure to alcohol vapors. Human volunteers exposed to concentrations of 0.7 to 1 percent ethyl alcohol vapors observed that the smell of alcohol was at first unbearable, although less unpleasant later, and that the eyes began to burn with increasing intensity after several minutes. This discomfort remained for the remainder of the exposure, which lasted for more than an hour, but no subsequent disturbances of the eyes were noted. A vapor concentration of 0.25 percent had no notable effect on the eyes.

FIRE EXTINGUISHERS

The fluid in fire extinguishers may be chlorobromomethane or tetrachloroethylene. Some water-filled extinguishers contain sulfuric acid; dry type fire extinguishers contain free-flowing powdered sodium or potassium bicarbonate. Fire-extinguishing foams are aggregates of small bubbles of gas made by mixing or agitation of air with water containing the foaming ingredients or by chemical reaction between aluminum sulfate and sodium bicarbonate to generate carbon dioxide.

Superficial injury of the eye has been observed from chloro-bromomethane and tetrachloroethylene. Sodium bicarbonate produced no damage in animal experiments when applied continuously over a 3-hour period; it is reasonable to expect similar effects from potassium bicarbonate, since the pH values are comparable.

FORMALDEHYDE

Formaldehyde is a gas in its natural state. It has a pungent suffocating odor. Commercially it is usually supplied as formalin, a 37 percent solution in water, or in solution in various organic solvents. Soluble in water and alcohol, it is used in urea, insulation, plastics, resins, ethylene glycol, fertilizer, dyes, medicine, embalming fluids, pre-servatives, and hardening agents.

Gaseous formaldehyde in the air is intensely irritating to the eyes and respiratory tract; therefore, damage of the eyes is not observed because the immediate discomfort it produces causes protective closure of the eyes. Aqueous solutions of formaldehyde splashed or dropped on human eyes have caused injuries ranging from severe permanent corneal opacification and loss of vision to minor transient injury or discomfort, depending on the concentrations of the solution. Even the most con-centrated commercial solution takes several minutes to produce a faint clouding of the epithelium. Early injury of the corneal stroma is marked by the denaturation and histologic fixing action of formaldehyde, which reduces the swelling potential of the stroma and masks the severity of injury until later, when infiltration and rejection of the devitalized tissue occur. A splash of a 40 percent solution in human eyes is immediately painful but characteristically leaves the eye looking deceptively normal for at least an hour or two after exposure, seemingly little injured; in the course of the next 12 hours all layers of the cornea may show obvious damage and edema, and the anterior segment may subsequently undergo devastating degeneration. Corneal hypesthesia and pericorneal ischemia seem to be particularly bad prognostic signs.

HYDROFLUORIC ACID

Hydrofluoric acid acts differently from all other acids, and onset of injury is insidious. Hydrofluoric acid is a solution of hydrogen fluoride in water. Both the gas and the liquid are extremely poisonous and injurious. The damage produced in the eye is far more extensive than that produced by the stronger halogen acids — hydroiodic, hydrobromic, and hydrochloric. The pH effects of the hydrofluoric acid appear to be minimally responsible for the damage observed; hydrochloric acid at the same pH causes damage to only the most superficial structures of the eye. Unlike the chloride from hydrochloric acid, the fluoride ion has a severe toxicity of its own, due in part to its ability to penetrate to deeper tissue layers and produce liquefaction necrosis.

Contact with both gaseous or liquid hydrofluoric acid produces immediate excruciating pain, irritation to the conjunctiva, bleeding lesions, and destruction of corneal epithelium with permanent scarring and blindness.

ISOPROPYL ALCOHOL

Isopropyl alcohol is somewhat less volatile than ethyl alcohol and more toxic on ingestion but has similar uses as a solvent, local antiseptic, and ingredient in cosmetics. The term is not interchangeable with rubbing alcohol; although most contain isopropyl alcohol, some brands contain only ethanol. Other names for isopropyl alcohol include isopropanol, dimethyl carbinol, secondary propyl alcohol, propan-2-ol, and alcohol isopropylicum.

Accidental splash contact with no immediate irrigation or exposure to high concentrations of isopropanol vapor have produced ragged abrasions of the corneal epithelium, which has been lost in patches. Corneal haziness, inflammation of the conjunctiva, and erythema of the eyelids have occurred. One case reported healing within 3 days. Tests run on rabbits' eyes have caused mild transitory injury graded 4 on a scale of 1 to 10 after 24 hours.

METHYL ALCOHOL

Methyl alcohol (methanol, wood alcohol, wood spirits) is a clear liquid soluble in water, alcohol, and ether. It is a widely used solvent in paints, varnishes, shellacs, and antifreeze fluid and with ethanol as a solid canned fuel (Sterno).

Methyl alcohol is an eye irritant. Direct contact with the eye produces a mild, reversible irritation, assuming treatment is initiated promptly. External eye contact has been alleged to have caused corneal opacities, but this appears to be the exception rather than the rule. Tests on rabbit eyes indicate that danger is slight. After application of a drop, a mild reversible reaction has been observed after 24 hours. No poisonous effects on the retina or optic nerve are observed after a drop of methanol on the eyes. One case has been reported where eye contact with chloroform and methyl alcohol was treated with immediate irrigation. After a period of very brief irritation, the patient had photophobia, persistent hyperemia, and staining of the cornea for a month's duration.

METHYLETHYL KETONE

A colorless liquid with an acetonelike odor, methylethyl ketone is used as a solvent in paint removers, cements, adhesives, cleaning fluids, and printing chemicals. Testing on rabbit eyes showed moderate reversible injury, graded 5 on a scale of 1 to 10. Warnings from the odor and irritation of the eyes and nose prevents exposure to vapor concentrations, which would induce narcosis similar to the systemic toxicity of acetone. Injury to the eyes has been produced in extreme conditions in animal experiments, where corneas became opaque but healed in 8 days spontaneously.

METHYLETHYL KETONE PEROXIDE

Methylethyl ketone peroxide is available as a 60 percent solution in dimethyl phthalate (Lupersol DDM) to serve as a catalyst for polymerizing plastics. The mixture has a high toxicity rating by ingestion. It is similar to hydrogen peroxide in that it readily releases oxygen. Experimentally a 40 percent solution has been found to cause severe damage to rabbit eyes. The maximum concentration that was not appreciably irritating to the eyes was 0.6 percent. Washing the eyes with water within 4 seconds after contact prevented injury of the eye in all cases.

OIL OF MUSTARD (ALLYL ISOTHIOCYANATE)

The volatile oil prepared from mustard seed is colorless or pale yellow with a pungent odor and acrid taste. It is present in black mustard seed and in horseradish. It has also been added to certain plastic glues or cements to discourage abuse by inhalation.

Exposure to oil of mustard externally causes burning and blistering of the skin, with ulceration on prolonged contact. The irritation is thought to arise from the reaction of the chemical with sulfhydryl groups on nerve endings in the eye tissue. The effects of the vapor on the eye include tearing and the development of keratitis, recovery from which is spontaneous but reportedly slow. In splash contact, the symptoms of one case history were red and swollen conjunctiva and lids and delayed clouding of the cornea that returned to normal in 6 to 7 days.

PETROLEUM PRODUCTS

Crude petroleum consists of a mixture of hydrocarbons of greatly varying molecular weight and structure, from which products such as gasoline, kerosene, naphtha, paraffin oil, petroleum ether, and benzine can be extracted.

Acute effects of the various liquid hydrocarbons of petroleum cause little or no injury on direct external contact with the eye. Kerosene, Deo-Base, Stoddard Solvent, and petroleum oil on rabbit and human corneas are essentially innocuous. More volatile derivatives such as high-test gasoline cause smarting and pain on splash contact with the eye but only slight transient corneal epithelial disturbance. Experimental exposure with animals indicated gasoline-containing tetraethyl lead causes no more injury than plain gasoline. Chronic effects include a detectable sense of irritation of the eyes and throat, which are perceived by human subjects with gasoline vapors in high concentrations in the air before any physical symptoms of irritation such as conjunctival hyperemia are visible. In workers chronically exposed in the petroleum industry abroad, there is said to be a related irreversible gradual loss of corneal and conjunctival sensitivity.

PHENOL

Phenol, also known as carbolic acid, phenic acid, or phenylic acid, is a colorless crystalline substance having a characteristic odor and caustic properties. Phenol and related substances rapidly denature all proteins they come in contact with. In dilute aqueous solution it has been used as an antiseptic and topical anesthetic, although in concentrated solutions it has caused second- or third-degree burns of the skin and systemic symptoms from percutaneous absorption. Acute effects of concentrated phenol have had severe consequences on human eyes, characteristically increasing lymph production in the conjunctiva and leaving the cornea white and hypesthetic. The eyelids become edematous and in some cases have been so severely damaged that plastic surgery was required. Severe iritis has been reported in at least one case. The final visual results have varied from complete recovery to partial recovery to blindness to loss of the eye.

SODIUM HYPOCHLORITE

Sodium hypochlorite is commonly available in aqueous solution, but it is rarely encountered as a solid because of instability. It is widely employed as a liquid bleach and antiseptic. Household laundry bleaches under various names such as Purex, Clorox, and Dazzle usually are approximately 5 percent solutions with pH adjusted to range of 10.5 to 12.5. Commercial laundry bleach, known as caustic soda bleach, contains 15 percent sodium hypochlorite at a pH slightly over 11.

Very few human eye injuries have been reported, presumably because most accidental splashes in the eye have been with the weaker 5 percent household solutions, and recovery has been rapid and complete. The more concentrated 15 percent solutions used in commercial laundries as a bleaching agent and in swimming pools as a disinfectant can be expected to cause more serious injury from a splash in the eye if the eye is not promptly irrigated with water. With irrigation, experimental evidence with rabbits shows that immediate pain suggests slight corneal epithelial haze and a conjunctival edema may develop and will return to normal in 24 to 48 hours. When the eye is not irrigated, a larger degree of corneal and conjunctival edema may develop with small hemorrhages, plus the rapid onset of a ground-glass appearance of the corneal epithelium. Such eyes have been observed to heal in 2 to 3 weeks with slight or no residual damage, although there has been neovascularization of the conjunctiva.

TEAR GAS AGENTS

Although loosely spoken of as a tear gas, these chemicals are actually white, crystalline powders dispersed as clouds of finely divided particles either by explosive cartridges or by pressurized solvent sprays (Mace). Chloracetophenone (CN Gas) is the agent most often identified as producing injurious effects; O-chlorobenzylidene malonitrile (CS Gas) has also caused eye damage. These chemicals combine with sulfhydryl groups in eye tissue to inactivate proteins and enzymes needed for sensory nerve activity. In weapons such as Mace, most of the solvent evaporates from the droplets, leaving chloracetophenone much more concentrated than the 1 percent in the original mixture. A third chemical, chloropicrin, produces strong irritation in the upper respiratory tract and to the skin. Vomiting often accompanies profuse lacrimation.

The body's primary defense is tearing, which may last 30 minutes or less. Laryngospasm may occur in response to the irritant effects. At low concentrations in the air the explosive-type tear gas causes much discomfort and blepharospasm, usually without injury to the cornea. In more direct contact, damage has occurred in the corneal endothelium, causing bluish corneal edema and wrinkling of the posterior surface of the cornea. Recovery has occurred in cases when the cornea was not opacified by other than transient edema. Exploded at close range, injuries have been serious enough to require complete removal of the eye. Cartridges stored for long periods may discharge the chemical in solid lumps rather than as a fine aerosol, causing added mechanical damage. With the spray type, initial symptoms of intense stinging and burning sensation in the eyes, tearing, spasm, and involuntary closure of the eyelids, irritation and watering of the nose, and burning of the skin are reported. In a study of 12 people sprayed with tear gas and not allowed to wash their eyes out, most injuries healed within 3 days. Two people suffered keratopathy uncorrectable by surgery for months beyond the original accident.

TOLUENE AND XYLENE (AROMATIC HYDROCARBONS)

Toluene is a flammable liquid with a benzenelike odor. It is employed in great quantities in chemical manufacture and as a solvent. It is commonly available to the public in airplane glue and some high-octane gasolines. It is also known as toluol, methyl-benzene, and phenyl methane. Xylene is a colorless liquid that has the odor characteristic of other aromatic hydrocarbons. Xylene is commonly found in paints, degreasers, and insecticides as a solvent; it is also used in protective coatings and aviation gasoline. It is also known as xylol and dimethyl benzene.

The literature describes moderate conjunctival hyperemia and corneal epithelial edema from exposure of human eyes to toluene. Despite a delay in irrigation for 4 to 5 minutes, the eyes returned to normal within 2 days. High concentrations of toluene vapor have been linked to dilation of the pupils, impairment of reaction, and slight pallor of the fundi. Accidental splash contamination of xylene in laboratory experiments on rabbits causes immediate discomfort and involuntary contraction of the eye muscle. Hyperemia of the conjunctiva and slight transient injury of the corneal epithelium also occurs. Such contact in human eyes has caused transient superficial damage with rapid recovery. Liquid xylene can cause irritation and noticeable vasodilation to the skin around the eyes. High concentrations of xylene vapor have caused considerable irritation, "foggy" vision, and vacuolar keratopathy.

TRICHLOROETHANE

Trichlorethane is available as two isomers; 1,1,1 trichloroethane (methyl chloroform, chlorothene) and 1,1,2 trichloroethane (vinyl trichloride). Both are moderately volatile and insoluble in water; 1,1,1 is widely used as a solvent and degreaser in many household products, including typewriter correction fluids, color film cleaners, insecticides, spot removers, fabric cleaning solutions, and paint removers.

Vapors at high concentrations are said to irritate the eyes. By splash or spray in the eyes, its injurious effect has been superficial and transient, resulting in chemosis and hyperemia. By inhalation, it appears to be one of the least toxic chlorinated aliphatic hydrocarbon solvents and has no known systemic toxic effect on the eye. Drop application of 1,1,1 to rabbit eyes caused conjunctival irritation but no corneal damage.

TRICHLOROETHYLENE

Trichloroethylene is a colorless, volatile liquid having a sweet odor similar to chloroform. The major industrial use is as a degreasing agent in dry cleaning. It is also found as an extraction solvent for fats and oils.

Direct contact of trichloroethylene with the eye may result in chemical burns of the lids, conjunctiva, and cornea. A splash or drop into the eye may cause a smarting pain and injuries to the corneal epithelium. Epithelium may be lost, but regeneration occurs. Complete spontaneous recovery is usually the case. Noninjurious exposure to low concentrations of trichloroethylene vapor has been reported to cause conjunctival irritation.

TURPENTINE OIL

Oil of turpentine is a volatile oil distilled from oleoresin or gum of various pine trees. There are four different types of turpentine (or grades) depending on the method of extraction and the distillation process. Toxicologically, they are essentially the same. A colorless liquid having a readily identifiable odor, turpentine is employed in paints and as a solvent for varnishes, lacquers, rubber, insecticides, synthetic camphor, medicinal liniment, wax-based polishes, and perfumes. Turpentine is mostly composed of terpene, an aromatic hydrocarbon. Volatile oils are also called essential oils, ethereal oils, and nondrying oils. Many or most of them have a high percentage of aromatic hydrocarbons combined with various esters aldehydes, and other organic compounds. They all behave in a similar manner.

Immediate severe pain and blepharospasm are reported after an accidental splash in the eye. This can be followed by conjunctival hyperemia and slight transient injury of the corneal epithelium. Temporary erosion of the epithelium can occur in severe cases, but no damage to the corneal stroma has been noted in human beings or animals after splash contact.

References — Chapter 22

A. J. Finkel, A. Hamilton, and H. L. Hardy, *Industrial Toxicology*, 4th ed. (Boston: John Wright, PSG, 1983).

W. M. Grant, *Toxicology of the Eye*, 2nd ed. (Springfield, IL: Charles C. Thomas, 1974).

W. M. Grant, *Toxicology of the Eye*, 3rd ed., (Springfield, IL: Charles C. Thomas, 1986).

M. Grayson, ed., *Kirk-Othmer Concise Encyclopedia of Chemical Technology*, 3rd ed. (New York: John Wiley & Sons, 1985).

M. M. Key, et al., *Occupational Diseases — A Guide to Their Recognition.* (Washington, DC: U.S. Dept. Health, Education and Welfare, PHS, CDC, NIOSH, 1977).

Merk Index, 10th ed. (Rahway, NJ: Merck and Company, 1983).

N. I. Sax, *Dangerous Properties of Industrial Materials*, 5th ed. (New York: Van Nostrand Reinhold 1979).

M. Sittig, *Handbook of Toxic and Hazardous Chemicals and Carcinogens*, 2nd ed. (New Jersey: Noyes Publications, 1985).

I. Skeist, *Handbook of Adhesives*, 2nd ed. (New York: Van Nostrand Reinhold, 1977).

P A R T   F I V E

LEGAL ASPECTS

Legal aspects of treating the poisoned patient are complex and, in many cases, unprecedented. New laws such as "right to know" legislation will have an enormous impact on the exposure of workers to toxic substances. Even regional poison control centers, apart from scant, legal constraints, are guided only by voluntary adherence to standards of the American Association of Poison Control Centers.

In such an "untested" environment, the following chapter is only a brief introduction to some of the basic concepts involved in fulfilling the health care professional's "duty of care" to a patient involved in a poisoning.

CHAPTER 23 LEGAL ASPECTS OF CLINICAL TOXICOLOGY

Health care professionals caring for intoxicated patients have several legal responsibilities. First, and foremost, they must exercise proper skill and care in the diagnosis and treatment of the patient. Second, they must comply with the reporting requirements of legislation when applicable. They should also take proper steps to help the patient in a possible lawsuit against third parties and to aid the state in prosecuting intentional poisoning and in enforcing laws regulating hazardous substances. Finally, the health care professional's duty to the public at large requires constant and aggressive efforts in the understanding and prevention of intoxication, acute and chronic, accidental and intentional, and specific and environmental.

PRIMARY DUTY TO THE PATIENT: PHYSICIAN'S LIABILITY

In the diagnosis and treatment of intoxication, as with other diseases, each member of the health care team must possess and exercise the degree of skill and learning ordinarily possessed and exercised under similar circumstances by the members of the profession in good standing. Each member must also use reasonable care and diligence and best judgment in applying skills to each case. Failure to possess the requisite skill or to exercise the requisite care, diligence, and best judgment, leading to patient injury, constitutes negligence or malpractice.

Intoxications are often emergencies. Fast decisions are usually required. Furthermore, since a good history may be impossible to obtain, proper treatment may be often delayed because the intoxicating agent is not readily known. All these factors enter into determining the proper standard of care against which a physician's handling of a patient is measured. Physicians should remember that in most cases the law presumes that they have acted with reasonable care and skill. Therefore, any patient claiming that the physician has acted negligently must prove the alleged negligence.* Physicians should not be frozen into inaction or

---

*There have been some cases of res ipsa loquitur against physicians. In these cases negligence is inferred and does not have to be proved. A leading care of res ipsa loquitur in malpractice is Ybarra v. Spangard, 93 Cal. App. 2d 43, 208 p. 2d 445.

unduly fear incorrect diagnosis and treatment. The law does not require that physicians ensure the *correctness* of their diagnosis and treatment, only that they use proper skill and diligence and their best judgment in diagnosis and treatment.

Increased liability is imposed on specialists and on specialized centers. If there has been a holding out of special knowledge and skill, then a higher degree of skill and care is required. Emergency room physicians, physicians specialized in toxicology, and emergency centers in general are bound to provide more than the average degree of skill and care provided by a general practitioner in a solo practice. The question of when a physician becomes a specialist or an institution a specialized center of toxicology is a question of fact, not a question of law. Some of the factors that may enter into this determination are specialized training of personnel, existence of a poison control center, wide laboratory resources, and a general accessibility of special knowledge and skill.

In cases of intoxication, consultation with other sources is common, for example, for identification of a substance, antidotes, and so forth. When consultation services are used, remember that the attending physician remains primarily liable and must use his or her best judgment in obtaining, evaluating, and applying information requested.

In addition to direct medical care, intoxication cases may require the health care professional to perform other duties. Intoxications may be accidental or intentional. If accidental, the causal chain of events and of the patients' home environment may require investigation. Detection of signs of patients' personal or social disorder (e.g., in cases of chronic intoxication such as alcoholism and cases of attempted suicide) with follow-up study or referral to appropriate specialists or social welfare agencies may in some cases be considered part of the physician's primary duty. In many situations the physician also must report to the proper authorities. If the intoxication is caused by food ingested at a public place, the physician must report to the local health authorities. If the patient is a child and parental abuse or neglect is suspected, reporting and referral provisions of local child abuse legislation must be complied with. If a homicidal poisoning is suspected, full reporting in the interest not only of the state but also of the patient is necessary. However, in the case of self-intoxication by illegal drugs or attempted suicide, the duty to report is overridden by the duty of confidentiality to the patient; the physician is in these situations protected by the physician-patient privilege.

SECONDARY DUTY TO PATIENT AND STATE

In the preceding section we have considered the duties owed by physicians and other health care personnel to their patients and instances of mandatory reporting. Breach of these duties may result in imposition of liability. In this section we will touch on other duties to the patient and to the state, the breach of which does not result in liability.

A patient who has been injured as a result of a negligent or intentional act of third parties may have some remedy against those parties. The state has an interest in prosecution of criminal acts. The physician should try to help the patient in the process of allocating liability for his or her injury and the state in successful prosecution. If a poisonous substance was not properly labeled and was accidentally ingested, the patient may have several lawsuits against those handling the substance. The state wants to prevent violation of labeling laws. If a contaminated restaurant meal causes a patient to become seriously ill, the patient may recover damages from that restaurant. The authorities want compliance with public health laws. If a patient has a prescription for a medicine, and the pharmacy fills that prescription with the wrong drug, causing the patient to suffer injury, the pharmacist or drug manufacturer may be liable to the patient. The state will seek compliance with the various laws that regulate the manufacture and sale of drugs.

In intoxication cases, the state has an interest in prosecution and the patient has numerous and varied potential lawsuits. In pursuing these actions, accurate record keeping and careful preservation of physical evidence will be extremely helpful to the patient, the state, and the attorneys involved. When the medical history is taken, the patients' own statements, given to the physician soon after the intoxication episode for the purpose of obtaining diagnosis and treatment, should be carefully recorded. These spontaneous statements, if of probative value, are admissible evidence in future lawsuits. In general, entries on all medical records about clinical and laboratory findings, extent of patients' injury, course of illness, and so forth should be clearly and timely made by professional personnel with firsthand knowledge of the facts recorded. Good records will also be most valuable to the physician required to testify at trial.

Physical evidence that may be pertinent to potential causes of action should be preserved. The physician should ensure that specimens, bottles, containers, and so forth are not lost, contaminated, spoiled, or damaged. Steps should also be taken for establishing a clear chain of custody of that evidence. Many times a piece of evidence of high probative value has been lost or has not been admitted at trial because it has been damaged while at the hospital or because an unexplained temporary misplacement has broken the necessary chain of custody.

DUTIES TO THE PUBLIC

In addition to directly caring for patients and helping with state prosecution and with patients' potential lawsuits against third parties, health care professionals dealing with intoxication have duties to the public at large. These duties include familiarity with legislation and governmental agencies in the area of toxicology and effects in poison prevention and public education.

Although thorough knowledge of legislation in the field is desirable, at least a working knowledge of major legislative efforts and of the related agencies should be expected. The input of physicians who deal firsthand with the injurious consequences of various substances is instrumental in achieving better legislation and better enforcement.

At the federal level, many laws regulate the quality and distribution of various substances. Of these the Federal Food, Drug, and Cosmetic Act is very important. It prohibits the manufacture, introduction, delivery, and receipt into interstate commerce of any food, drug, device, or cosmetic that is adulterated or misbranded as well as the act of adulteration or misbranding. The Poison Prevention Packaging Act of 1970 provides for special packaging of certain dangerous substances and is particularly important in cases of accidental intoxication of children. The Fair Packaging and Labeling Act prevents use of unfair or deceptive methods of packaging and labeling of certain products. The Federal Hazardous Substances Act prohibits the interstate shipment of misbranded or inadequately labeled substances that are suitable or intended for household use.

Familiarity with legislation should be followed by maintenance of regular channels of communication and active cooperation with enforcing agencies. The Department of Health, Education, and Welfare in general and especially the Food and Drug Administration have wide responsibilities in regulating hazardous substances. The Department of Agriculture and the Department of the Interior regulate pesticides and some pollution problems. Pollution is specifically handled by the Environmental Protection Agency. The Department of Justice, through the Bureau of Narcotics and Dangerous Drugs, controls the sale, distribution, and possession of such substances. It is important to keep a file of the publications of these agencies, those intended for physicians and other health care personnel as well as those intended for the general public.

Distribution of health education material can be most effective when received at the time of the intoxication episode. Physicians should not only be informed of the latest regulatory developments but should also help enforcement by reporting to the agencies their observation and findings, making suggestions for possible agency action, and cooperating with the health education programs of the various agencies.

Although there has been considerable activity in the control of dangerous substances at the federal level, familiarity and active cooperation with state and local health authorities are vital. The physician must remember that states are primarily responsible for the health of their residents. Fast and effective solutions to a specific problem are usually found at the state and local levels.

In addition to governmental sources, the physician handling episodes of intoxication must use other community resources. Among such resources, crisis intervention services such as suicide and child abuse hot lines and Acid Rescue may prove helpful in the management of an intoxication.

POISON CONTROL CENTERS

In the past few years poison control centers have been established throughout the United States. The functioning of poison control centers is described in Chapter 24.

Since poison control centers are relatively new institutions performing a variety of functions, their legal status and potential liability are not fully determined. They may be treated as parts of a health institution if they are associated with these institutions. Basically a poison control center has these functions:

1. Keeps and provides on request information on various substances: composition, toxicity, antidotes, methods of therapy, and so forth. This information in varying degrees is available to physicians, emergency centers, and the public at large.

2. Compiles and reports data for the purpose of enforcement of legislation and research in prevention of intoxication.

3. Educates the public in poison prevention.

Of these general functions, the one that presents some possibilities of imposition of liability is the function of providing information for the purpose of diagnosis and treatment of intoxication. Although no action brought against a poison control center has been successful, the potential for liability is nevertheless present. The center must keep its files and library complete and current and must employ adequately trained personnel. The fact that often no remuneration is received by the poison center for its services should not be considered a shield against liability. The rule that gratuitousness of services does not prevent imposition of liability against a physician who has undertaken to treat a patient and has been negligent may be extended to poison centers. If the center has held out to the public that it will provide to those seeking it accurate information by trained personnel on a 24-hour-a-day basis, a person who is injured as a result of inaccurate or misleading information received from a poison control center may attempt to bring an action against the center on the basis of negligence, implied contract, or warranty theories.

Therefore, a center must fulfill promises made to the public. It must also keep accurate records. Every request for information must be timely, recorded with as much data as possible on the caller and on the information and advice given by the center. All entries must include date and time and must be signed or initialed by the personnel who handled the request.

At present, poison control centers, as simple providers of information to parties who are often anonymous, have not been held liable for injuries related to allegedly faulty information given. However, continued avoidance of liability will only be ensured by high standards of accuracy in the poison files, well-trained, round-the-clock personnel, and clear, complete, and timely records.

In addition to the direct duty to the person seeking information, poison control centers must fulfill their duty of reporting to help enforce existing legislation and generate new, needed legislative activity. Although reporting is largely accomplished through the National Clearing House for Poison Control Centers, additional reporting to other agencies may be helpful. Reporting of obvious violations of, for example, the Federal Food, Drug, and Cosmetic Act (e.g., contaminated foods, misbranding) and the Federal Hazardous Substance Act (failure to label dangerous substances accordingly) will cause quick and effective law enforcement. Reporting could cause revision and development of new regulations. For example, if a container that has satisfied agency standards for implementation of the Poison Prevention Packaging Act is repeatedly found to be involved in accidental poisoning in children, reporting may cause not only product recall but also revision of that standard.

Public education activities of the poison control center should not only involve individual, home, and environmental prevention measures but should also educate the public about existing protective legislation.

CONCLUSION

The legal principles governing health care professionals and health centers should be an integral part of the education of physicians and other health care personnel. In handling intoxications, health care professionals must be aware of the various duties they owe to the patient, the state, and the public at large. Familiarity with the legal consequences of their acts in diagnosis and treatment, in record keeping, in reporting, and in giving out information will enable health care professionals to give better and more complete care and will also help them avoid unwanted and vexatious litigation. The health care professional in toxicology must also be aware of the large-picture legislation regulating various substances and jurisdiction and work of pertinent local, state, and federal agencies so that they may use their knowledge, expertise, and firsthand observations to promote effective legislation and public education for the prevention of intoxication.

References — Chapter 23

Anderson, "Physicians' Testimony — Hearsay Evidence or Expert Opinion: A Question of Professional Competence," 53 *Tex. L. Rev.* 296-322 (1975).

Ficarra, "The Hospital Emergency Room and the Law," 12 *Calif. W. J. Rev.* 223-36 (1976).

Fisher, "Federal/State Concurrent Regulations," 29 *Food Drug Cosm. L. J.* 20-26 (1974).

A. R. Gough, K. M. Healey, and S. R. Rupp, "Poison Control Centers, From Aspirin to PCBs and the Scarlet Runner Bean: A Study of Legal Anomaly and Social Necessity." *Santa Clara Law Review* 23:791-809, 1983.

Merrill, "Compensation for Prescription Drug Injuries," 59 *Va. L. Rev.* 1-120 (1973).

Pfeifer, "Section 305 Hearings and Criminal Prosecutions," 31 *Food Drug Cosm. L. J.* 376-81 (1976).

Rodwin, "A Violation of the Federal Food Drug and Cosmetic Act — A Crime in Search of a Criminal," 31 *Food, Drug Cosm. L. J.* 616-26(1976).

Tondell and Chittenden, "Work of the Medical Profession Liability Commission," 62 *A.B.A.J.* 1580-4 (1976).

Tracy, "Emergency Care: Physicians Should be Placed Under an Affirmative Duty to Render Essential Medical Care in Emergency Circumstances," 7 *U.C.D.L.* Rev. 246-79 (1974).

THE REGIONAL POISON CENTER: A 'SYSTEMS' APPROACH

Poisoning is a medical condition that demands a systems approach because of the nature of the poisoning incident itself. It has a sudden onset; it is potentially life threatening; it occurs in unpredictable locations outside of hospital settings; there are time constraints for treatment to prevent death; and there is a necessity for successive treatment and triage in multiple locations by multiple providers. When these characteristics exist for any medical condition, a system is necessary to guarantee the patient adequate care. The various personnel and resources must be coordinated into a planned response in which the patient's problem is identified and classified and he is selectively treated by telephone or routed to resources that meet his particular needs. Operational, treatment, and triage protocols under which the patient care providers operate are crucial to patient survival.

The focal point of the poison system's response, the regional poison center, is the subject of discussion in the next chapter. The center serves the region's public and professionals by providing telephone consultation and treatment or appropriate referral to a treatment center. The regional center provides a source of cumulative expertise within the region. The experience and data of all the health care providers who manage poisonings are collected at the regional center. If the center coordinates effectively with other regional centers, it then provides to its region the accumulated expertise of the nation.

CHAPTER 24 THE REGIONAL POISON CENTER

Since the early 1950s poison control centers have demonstrated their importance in treating accidental ingestion. At this time there are over 500 poison centers still registered in the United States and its possessions. These centers provide a variety of services, and most centers supply some information to the public. However, most of these "traditional" poison control centers are located directly in, and are operated by, emergency room departments and their staff. More recently, *regional* poison centers have finally become a reality, and in 1982 the Criteria for Designation of Regional Centers was formulated by the American Association of Poison Control Centers (AAPCC). In adapting to these criteria in the 1980s, regional centers have become an indispensable part of the emergency care delivery system. Among the key features of regional centers is the geographic region that is specified in conjunction with state authorities and local health agencies and the interaction between the poison information center and the poison treatment centers in a given region. A typical regional poison prevention and treatment program provides the following:

1. Poison information and consultation
2. Emergency treatment
3. Emergency public access, utilizing toll-free telephone system and direct link to 911 for
    a. Information
    b. Treatment
    c. Follow-up
    d. Referral
4. Professional education
5. Coordination of interhospital transport of poisoned patients
6. Data collection and evaluation
7. Research/quality control
8. Public education/poison prevention teaching
9. Regional Emergency Medical Services/poison system development

Although participation in the AAPCC regional certification process is voluntary, to be designated a "regional" center the following specific services must be available to provide adequate information and consultation:

- The regional poison control service must be capable of providing *information* 24 hours a day, 365 days a year to both consumers and health care professionals.
- The regional poison control center shall be readily accessible by *telephone* from all areas within the region.
- The regional poison control center shall maintain comprehensive *poison information resources*.
- The regional poison control center shall maintain written *management protocols* for consumer calls that provide a consistent approach to evaluation and management of pre-hospital toxic exposures.
- *Staff* of the regional poison control center must consist of a medical director who is qualified and available to provide medical training and supervision of information specialists. Poison information specialists must be qualified to read, understand, and interpret standard poison information resources and to transmit that information in a logical, concise, and understandable way to both health care professionals and consumers, and to transmit standardized poison center treatment protocols approved by the medical director. This requirement is considered to be met if the person has a degree in or is qualified for licensure in nursing, pharmacy, or medicine (see Poison Center Staff later in this chapter).

ANSWERING POISON CALLS: TRIAGE FUNCTION OF A POISON CENTER

The following information is provided for those health care professionals routinely working in or with a poison center. As more regional centers interact with local emergency departments, it is important that personnel have some idea of the triage function and history-taking process of a poison center to save themselves and their patients time and improve efficiency.

The concept of providing lifesaving, timesaving and energy-saving information over all sorts of communication devices has become an integral and indispensable part of the health care delivery system in all industrialized nations. All sorts of patient health data can be communicated electronically from one place to virtually any other place in the time it takes to make a telephone call. About 95 percent of the population in the United States has 24-hour direct access to telephone communication of one kind or another. Thus, a "centrally" located information center within a given region can provide immediate information, first-aid assistance, treatment or referral direction, follow-up, and assurance, within seconds of a phone call. Within reasonable limits the population served (usually between 2 and 10 million persons) is not concerned about the geographic location of the information center. However, this emphasizes the importance of good interrelationships between the regional information center and local poison treatment facilities.

Since providing information over the telephone is one of the hallmarks of a poison center, it is important that the staff also be trained in history taking and triaging patients by telephone. Studies have demonstrated that telephone-trained nonphysician personnel in a given specialty are better providers of certain types of information than untrained physicians providing the same information.

When communicating instructions, the call taker should attempt to be as clear and concise as possible. If instructions are given, it is best to advise the caller to write down the instructions and then read them to the call taker. Using this method minimizes misunderstandings.

Remember that although the information may be familiar to the call taker, it is probably not familiar to the caller. Facts and data regarding toxicologic information have little relevance to someone unfamiliar with them. However, interpreting the data in a statement that is understandable to a nonmedical person is very useful in emphasizing the seriousness or lack of seriousness of a situation. For example, if a parent calls and states that his or her 25-lb, 2-year-old child has just ingested 5 baby aspirin (1 1/4 grain), rather than simply stating "it won't hurt the child," the call taker should explain the relationship of toxicity to weight, give an indication of what might be a toxic amount for the child, and reassure the parent that with this ingestion there is no problem.

Even though the order of obtaining information varies with each call, it is best to determine initially what was ingested and whether the patient is symptomatic. Other important factors are the amount of substance ingested and the time elapsed since ingestion. Age, weight, history of prior illness, and establishing whether the contaminant is a solid, liquid, gas, powder, cream, tablet, or capsule are additional and necessary facts that should be elicited from the caller.

Once the suspected agent is identified, information regarding brand name and proper spelling, general use of the product, and, in the case of tablets and capsules, the coding or other markings is essential for determining the toxicity through available resources. In many cases the effectiveness of ingestion management will be based on the effectiveness with which the poison center staff investigates the ingestion incident.

The following lists may be helpful not only in trying to establish the amount ingested and helping the caller to arrive at an accurate evaluation of the toxic episode but also in initiating therapy.

PROCEDURES REGARDING THE TREATMENT OF SPECIFIC TYPES OF POISONING

The order of obtaining information in an emergency varies with each call. A suggested format is given below. Regional poison centers employ standard reporting forms to capture information quickly. The information on these standard forms is then submitted in various ways to the National Data Collection System of the American Association of Poison Control Centers.

RECEIVING THE CALL

1. Calm the caller. Fewer exaggerations occur when the caller is in control of the situation. Offer reassurance as early as possible.

2. Determine *what* was ingested, sprayed, or spilled on the skin or in the eye(s), get qualifying details about the offending substance. Obtain specific brand name and spelling, or general type of product, coding or marking on tablet or capsule.

3. Determine if the contaminant is a solid, liquid, powder, cream, tablet or capsule, prescription item, over-the-counter.

4. Determine amount ingested. (See procedure below for role playing.)

5. Determine time since ingestion and record time of call.

6. Record any symptoms that have occurred since the time of the ingestion. Try not to suggest any during questioning, remaining compassionate but objective.

7. Record age (and weight of the patient if applicable to any dosage calculations which may be necessary).

8. Obtain phone number, put caller on "hold" only if necessary to research the problem. If possible stay on the line with the caller, offering continual reassurance while you assess the situation. If you expect the wait to be lengthy, suggest that the caller give the patient a drink of appropriate liquid, unless this is contraindicated by the product ingested or any symptoms present.

9. Research the problem. Know where to look.

10. Make the decision for observation, home treatment, or referral to a health care facility.

Ingestions

Liquids. For the most part, callers tend to exaggerate when estimating quantities, especially when liquids are involved, but the following considerations may be useful.

      1. Determine the quantity of the product in the container when it was purchased. If the caller has the original container, he or she can check the label for this information.

      2. In most cases, at least a small portion had been used before the ingestion episode. A somewhat vague estimation of amount may be obtained by inquiring whether the container was about three fourths, one half, or one fourth full before ingestion. For a more accurate assessment of content, instruct the caller to fill up the container to the preingestion level and then remove the amount suspected, using a measuring device to determine the quantity.

      3. When children ingest liquids, particularly those with containers that are difficult to manipulate, they frequently spill far more than they ingest. When spilling occurs, estimation of the ingested amount is not always possible and treatment relies more on the type of product and its toxicity.

      4. On occasion the scent of the product on the patient's breath may be rather pronounced. Absence of obvious odor, however, does not always indicate that ingestion has not occurred. Therefore, although this procedure is helpful in determining that something probably has been ingested, it should never be used to rule out ingestion.

Tablets or capsules. Flavored, sweetened, or sugar-coated tablets are among the most palatable and frequently ingested drugs by children. It is entirely possible for most children to consume large quantities of these agents, since their taste may resemble that of candy. This is in contrast to those drugs that are unflavored, which are usually ingested in much smaller quantities.

      In most situations, however, the amount of tablets or capsules ingested is not easily determined and the ingestion must be related to the individual agent's toxicity. When the ingestion of tablets or capsules is involved, the following process is useful if a definite amount cannot be determined.

      1. If an over-the-counter product is ingested and the original container is available, the number of tablets or capsules when purchased should be listed on the label. The number previously used and the number remaining can be estimated.

2. For prescription drugs, if the original amount cannot be determined, the prescription number and name of the pharmacy may be obtained from the label and the pharmacy called to establish the amount. After the original number has been obtained, ask the caller how many tablets or capsules were to be taken each day and for how many days they have been taken. With both over-the-counter and prescription drugs, subtracting the number remaining from the amount estimated to be present before the incident will give the approximate number ingested.

3. Other considerations regarding tablets and capsules include whether any may have fallen on the floor and whether the child possibly placed them somewhere out of sight. Many times parents call a poison center only to find afterward that the substance in question was simply misplaced.

The following procedures suggest an order for taking information from a caller and present a sort of verbal "volley" that is useful in obtaining facts in an emergency. These procedures may be adapted to a clinician taking a history from a parent of a patient in an emergency department, or a paramedic investigating an ingestion in the field.

DETERMINING AMOUNT INGESTED

Find out if the product ingested was a liquid, powder, or cream, a tablet or capsule, or a solid. Then refer to the following. As a help in determining the amount ingested and to facilitate role playing before triaging an actual emergency, the following is in "caller says/your response" format:

Liquids, Powders, or Creams

(e.g., motor oil, liquid makeup, or powdered or liquid detergent)

The caller tells you . . .	You may respond or suggest the following . . .
"He didn't get much." or "He only took a little."	"Was it closer to a few drops, a teaspoonful, or a tablespoonful?" If the caller does not know, go on to the series of questions below: "How much did the container have in it

when purchased? That is, how many ounces, etc.?"

If the caller still has the container, this information can be found on the label.

"I don't know how much he took."

"Did you use any of it, or was it full?"

If the caller says some has been used, ask if it had been almost full, about three fourths, one half, or one quarter full. From the answers to the above questions, estimate how much was in the container when the patient obtained it. Now continue with the questions below.

"How much is left in the container?"

If the container is not transparent, the caller can hold it up to a light to see the level of the contents. If it is impossible to see in this way (e.g., it if is in a can), the caller can pour out the remaining contents into a measuring cup, or into 8-oz glasses. Subtracting the amount left from the amount that was in the container when the patient obtained it will provide an estimate of the maximum amount that the patient could have ingested. However, children often spill products or spit them out. Asking the following questions may help to determine how much was actually ingested.

"Was any spilled on or around the patient?"

If possible, get the caller to estimate how much.

"Did he spit some out, or did he swallow all of the product?"

If the caller answers yes to spilling or spitting some of the product out, then the patient has ingested less than the original calculation.

"He may not have taken any."

Check around the mouth for signs of the product and determine if any odors are on the breath. If there are signs of the product in the patient's mouth, it may be established that an ingestion did occur. Even if there are no signs of the product, however, do not assume that the patient did not ingest the product.

Tablets or Capsules

(e.g., aspirin, vitamins, or birth control pills)

The caller tells you ...	You may respond or suggest the following ...
"He didn't get many." or "He only took a few."	"Exactly how many did he take?" If the caller does not know, go on to the series of questions below.
"I don't know how many he took."	"How many did the bottle contain originally, when it was purchased?" If the caller still has the container, this information should be on the label of the product. If it's not available, an estimate will have to be made. If it is a prescription drug and the caller does not know how many tablets were in the container, ask how many were to be taken each day and for how many days the tablets were to be taken. If the caller cannot furnish this information, contact the pharmacy that filled the prescription.
	"How many have you taken since you bought them?" If it is a prescription or other daily medicine, ask how many were to be taken each day, and how many days had passed since the person started taking them. From the answers to the above questions, one can calculate about how many tablets were in the container when the patient obtained it. Then continue with the following questions.

"How many are left now?"
If one subtracts the number left from the number that were in the bottle, the answer is the maximum number that the patient could have ingested. However, people, especially children, often spill or misplace tablets. Ask the following questions to determine this.

"Did any fall on the floor, or roll under furniture?"
(Also check a child's diaper.)
If the caller says no, have him/her physically check to make sure. If the caller says yes, ask him/her to find and count any that were spilled. Subtract the number spilled from the maximum number the patient could have ingested to determine the number probably ingested.

"He may not have taken any."

"What makes you think he did take some?"
If the caller has a valid reason for believing that the patient did ingest some of the tablets, ask the series of questions from "I don't know how many he took."

Solids

(e.g., crayons, wax, or bar soap)

The caller tells you . . .	You may respond or suggest the following . . .
"He didn't get much." or "He only took a little."	"Can you judge how large a piece was eaten? Was it closer to 1/4-in square (about the size of a pea); 1/2-in square (about the size of a bouillon cube, sugar cube or marble); 1-in square (about the size of a ping pong ball or golf ball)." If the caller does not know, go on to the series of questions below.

"I don't know how much he took."

"How large was the product when you bought it?"
If the caller still has the container, this information may be listed on the package. If not, get an approximate size of the product (2 inches square, 1-in square, etc.)

"Have you used any of it, or was it all there?"
If the caller says some of it had been used, ask if most of it was left, or about three fourths, one half, or one fourth was left. From the answers to the above questions, you can estimate approximately how large the solid was when the patient obtained the product.

"How much is left now?"
Have the caller closely estimate how much is now left. If you subtract how much is now left from how much there was when the patient obtained it, you will have an estimate of the maximum amount the patient could have ingested.

"Did he spit some of the product out, or did he swallow it all?"

"Are there any pieces around that fell to the floor, or rolled under the furniture?"
If the caller answers yes to the above questions, you know the patient ingested less than the amount you originally calculated.

"He may not have taken any."

"Check the mouth for signs of the product and see if you can smell any odor of the product on the breath."
If there are signs of the product in the patient's mouth, you may be able to establish that an ingestion did occur. Even if there are no signs of the product, however, do not assume that the patient did not ingest the product.

Making a decision regarding treatment or referral following

an ingestion can be very difficult over the telephone. The above procedures merely suggest a format for obtaining as much information as possible in a short time. Since telephone histories surrounding ingestions are notoriously inaccurate, always lean toward having the patient seen in an emergency treatment facility when there is any question about the accuracy of the history. This is particularly true when known toxic drugs and chemicals are involved.

Eye Contaminants

    1. Advise immediate decontamination. Tell the caller to flood the eye with water or saline, depending on the patient's location. Time so outweighs other considerations that water, or any innocuous watery solution should be used at once. Do not waste time looking for a special irrigation fluid. (See Chap. 2, Emergency Treatment, and Chap. 22, Eye Contamination.)

    2. Locate information about the product or chemical contaminant while the caller is irrigating the eye.

    3. Consider the contaminant's toxicity, concentration, and quantity involved. Advise on further medical treatment. It is far better to err on the side of suggesting medical follow-up that may prove to be unnecessary than to do nothing and have latent damage appear afterward.

    The chart below shows the relationship of pH to potential for irritation of the mucous membranes and skin. A pH below 2.5 (very acid) and above 11 (very alkaline) is a good indication of potential chemical injury.

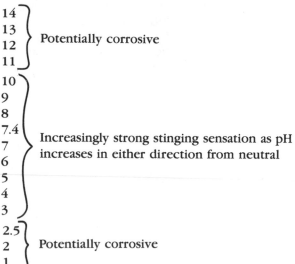

pH	
14 13 12 11	Potentially corrosive
10 9 8 7.4 7 6 5 4 3	Increasingly strong stinging sensation as pH increases in either direction from neutral
2.5 2 1	Potentially corrosive

Skin Contaminants

  1. Drench skin with water. Use the most readily available source (shower, hose, faucet, etc.).

  2. Apply a steady stream of water while removing person's clothing.

  3. Irrigate for 3 to 5 minutes for water-soluble substances and for at least 15 minutes for acids, alkalies, and all soluble irritants-corrosives.

  4. Any symptoms or signs of irritation that persist should be referred for treatment. See the chart on page 220 showing the relationship of pH to potential for skin and mucous membrane irritation. Further treatment to involved areas is the same as for thermal burns of a similar severity.

  Some chemicals have anesthetic properties (e.g., phenol). Do not rely on the absence of pain as an indicator for stopping irrigation with these chemicals. Tell the caller to flush thoroughly for the prescribed time.

Inhalations

  1. Take whatever steps necessary to remove the victim from exposure or provide adequate ventilation.

  2. Establish and maintain adequate airway.

  3. Suggest oxygen and artificial respiration if necessary.

  4. Identify the vapor or gas. Use a specific antidote when available (e.g., amyl nitrite for cyanide poisoning), followed by other components of the cyanide antidote kit or oxygen for carbon monoxide.

Envenomating Animals

Stinging insects (hymenoptera).

  1. If a stinger is present, remove it with a scraping action. Instruct the caller to be careful not to squeeze any additional venom into the skin when removing the stinger. Do not use a tweezer for this reason.

  2. Wash the skin with mild soap and water.

  3. Apply ice to the surface. A few hours of intermittent application is usually sufficient.

  4. Advise about the danger of an allergic reaction. Refer the patient if symptoms beyond a local reaction exist. See Chapter 18 for additional discussion.

Spiders.

1. Remember that spiders are arachnids, not insects. Treatment differs considerably. Two spiders are particularly dangerous to people, the black widow (*Latrodectus mactans*) and the brown recluse (*Loxosceles reclusa*).

2. Do *not* apply ice. In a brown recluse bite, this will aggravate local vasoconstriction.

3. Since considerable differential diagnosis (impetigo, herpes, and other infectious diseases) is necessary, refer the victim to a qualified physician.

Snakes. Snakebite is always cause for referral to a medical facility for evaluation. See Chapter 18 for protocols.

Food Poisoning

1. Ascertain the signs and symptoms — onset, severity, and duration.

2. Identify the suspected food, the method of preparation, and the type of storage.

3. Using poison center resources, determine the most likely organism or substance responsible.

4. If signs and symptoms are considered minimal, advise a clear liquid diet with a gradual progression to a regular diet.

5. If signs and symptoms are moderate to severe, refer for physician treatment to include differential diagnosis.

6. Emesis is not indicated unless a suspected contaminant has been ingested within a short period, usually 30 to 60 minutes.

7. If botulism (*Clostridium botulinum*) is suspected, refer immediately for medical treatment.

8. Notify the local health department. Appropriate laboratory support must be coordinated with the treating health care facility.

POISON CONTROL CENTER STAFF

For many years there were few established guidelines or controls and thus very little consistency among poison control centers. The number of potentially toxic substances and the body of knowledge and treatment regimens to deal with them have outpaced the ability of emergency and primary care health providers to retain or retrieve the necessary information and handle exposures unaided by specialty centers. These centers require a specialized staff whose full-time job involves providing management information to primary care practitioners.

A *regional* poison center must be maintained around the clock by a well-trained and well-supervised staff. The advantages of a full-time staff are twofold: (1) the personnel are initially trained in dealing with the problems of ingestion and (2) day-to-day exposure to the problem enhances the staff's knowledge and ability to cope with it effectively.

The staff qualifications should be as follows:

Medical director. The medical director should be qualified to provide medical training to and supervision of information specialists, to be responsible for medical decisions and treatment protocols, and to provide direct patient care, telephone supervision, or case consulting on the hospitalized poisoned patient either as the attending physician or as a consultant. The medical director should have specialty certification or board eligibility in pediatrics, emergency medicine, internal medicine, or another primary care specialty, plus training or experience in medical toxicology. One way of demonstrating qualifications is for the medical director to meet requirements of standing for the medical toxicology certification examination of the American Board of Medical Toxicology. The medical director should have a medical staff appointment at one or more comprehensive poison treatment facilities. Ideally, at least 50 percent of the medical director's time should be spent in poison center activities, especially in direct patient care, telephone supervision, or case consulting and in staff performance review.

Poison information specialists. Poison information specialists must be qualified to read, understand, and interpret standard poison information resources, to transmit that information in a logical, concise, and understandable way to both health care professionals and consumers, and to transmit standardized poison center treatment protocols approved by the medical director. This requirement would be considered to be met if the person has a degree or is qualified for licensure in nursing, pharmacy, or medicine or has equivalent training experience, plus training or experience in toxicology and poison information sciences. Poison information specialists should spend at least 20 hours a week in poison center-related activities including providing telephone consultation, teaching, or public education or in poison-center operations. Although they may be part-time staff or have a part-time assignment to the poison center, 100 percent of their time should be dedicated to poison-center activities while assigned to the center.

Other poison information providers. Other poison information providers must be qualified to read and understand standard poison information resources and to transmit that information understandably to both health care professionals and consumers under the supervision of a poison information specialist or the medical director. This requirement will be considered to be met if the person has an appropriate health care-oriented background and specific training or experience in poison information sciences. Although they may be part-time staff or have a part-time commitment to the poison center, 100 percent of their time should be dedicated to poison-center activities while assigned to the center.

Poison center specialty consultants. Poison-center specialty consultants should be qualified by training or experience to provide limited but highly sophisticated toxicology information or patient care for a specific area of toxicology. These consultants should be available on call with an expressed commitment to provide consultation services on an on-call, as-needed basis. The list of consultants should reflect the type of poisonings encountered in the region.

Administrative staff. Poison center administrative personnel should be qualified by training or experience to supervise finances, operations, personnel, data analysis, and other administrative functions. This position could be filled by medical director or a poison information specialist as part of the time that *is not* committed to direct consultative services or by other institutional personnel.

Education Staff

Professional education. Educational personnel should be qualified by training or experience to provide quality professional education lectures or materials to their peers or less sophisticated health care professionals. This role would generally be filled by the medical director or qualified poison information specialist.

Consumer education. Consumer educational personnel should be qualified by training or experience to provide consumer-oriented poison prevention or poison center awareness presentations. They must be capable of verbal presentations in front of consumer audiences and have sufficient understanding of the material to answer consumer questions accurately. They may be full-time, part-time, or volunteer staff.

The staff of the poison center should include physicians, nurses, and pharmacists. Employment of pharmacists along with a well-trained nursing staff offers many benefits in providing efficient information services. The pharmacist's basic knowledge of pharmacology and the nurse's human relationship training provide dimensions of care that neither professional can provide alone. A physician with toxicologic experience should direct all personnel and provide consultation service to other physicians who require it.

Usually a center in a large city or one encompassing a large geographic area has access to many manufacturers and public services, such as local, state, and federal agencies, universities, and other research institutions. These groups are often invaluable in lending their expertise in fields such as chemistry, botany, and zoology. It is absolutely essential for a regional center to establish a professional relationship with these organizations.

Poison Center Database

Each regional poison center is solely responsible for building, purchasing, or otherwise procuring its own technical information database. Most centers use microfiche systems (i.e., Poisindex® by Micromedex, Inc.) or the Computerized Clinical Information System (CCIS®, also by Micromedex, Inc.) on compact laser disk. Within the last few years these information systems have been supplying toxicologic information at a "state of the art" technologic pace. The following systems have been developed by and in conjunction with regional poison center personnel who are specialists in clinical toxicology, pharmacology, and emergency medicine.

Poisindex is a detailed toxicology database designed to identify and provide ingredient information on over 300,000 commercial, industrial, pharmaceutical, and botanical substances. The Poisindex system also provides detailed management and treatment protocols in the event of a toxicology problem due to ingestion, absorption, or inhalation of any of the substances listed. Poisindex is indexed by brand/trade name, manufacturer's name, generic/chemical name, street/slang terminology, botanical, and common name.

The *Drugdex System* is an up-to-date, unbiased, and referenced drug information system. It includes both drug evaluations and drug consultations on over 3,700 investigational and foreign, FDA-approved, and over- the-counter preparations. This system is indexed by U.S. and foreign brand/trade names, disease states, and drug information terms.

Emergindex, a system of diagnostics and therapeutics, is a referenced clinical information system designed to present pertinent medical data for the practice of acute care medicine. This system is divided into six major sections: clinical reviews, differential reviews, clinical abstracts, arrhythmia managements, prehospital care, and emergency and critical care techniques. The database is indexed with a 40,000 key-word medical thesaurus.

Tablet and capsule identification is usually accomplished with the *Identidex* System. It uses manufacturer imprint codes as the primary identification resource. Also included are color and physical description. The Identidex System contains over 23,000 entries and identification on U.S. and foreign ethical/prescription drugs, over-the-counter look-alike/rip-off drugs, and slang/street terms.

All the above systems can be purchased individually from Micromedex, Inc. The CCIS System mentioned above is a compilation of some or all Micromedex databases, Poisindex, Identidex, Drugdex, and Emergindex as well as drug and dosing calculation programs and toxicology nomograms into an efficient, computerized clinical information system. All these systems provide the user with group medical opinion and complete annotation, allowing for the most reliable and current information available to poison centers today. Although it is essential for a poison center to have and use these basic information systems, it is also important to maintain and use secondary and primary resources.

Secondary information resources are textbooks and compendia that present information by category or classification in such a way that clinical experience can be used to make general recommendations regarding treatment. A couple of examples are the now classic publications of *Clinical Toxicology of Commercial Products* by Gosselin et al. and *Handbook of Poisoning* by Robert Dreisbach.

Primary information resources are original journal articles reporting case studies, original research, clinical trials, and so on. A regional poison center should have access to those journals and publications known to be available in this field of interest, such as the *Journal of Toxicology* by Marcel Dekker and *Veterinary and Human Toxicology* published by the American Academy of Veterinary and Comparative Toxicology.

Of course there are many other toxicology information resources to be considered. Toxicology is a broad subject area, and it is economically impossible for a poison center to keep information on site for the many disciplines that are encompassed. Many poison centers have developed their own sophisticated on-site systems using computers or card files that augment the major toxicology database.

Communication among poison centers, patient treatment facilities, commercial technical databases, and industrial-electronic "bulletin boards" constitutes another important network of information exchange that may be vastly improved by use of electronic facsimile devices, telephone modems, and other technologic advancements. These devices can transmit information from one area to another using modified telephone equipment. Sending information by facsimile or modem eliminates the possibility of error that often results from verbal communication. Telephone modem communication with off-site databases such as the National Library of Medicine's MEDLARS (Medical Literature Analysis and Retrieval System) is becoming quite common without the use of intermediate search services formerly available only through medical libraries. Computerized poison centers can investigate the toxicity of foreign drugs; analytical data regarding carcinogenicity; ocular, inhalation, and skin toxicity; as well as many other toxicology-related subjects without ever leaving the poison center.

As information centers in an "information age," poison centers provide a very real and essential role as a clearing house for highly specialized and technical information. The development of the regional toxicology database is an ongoing challenge to provide primary health care providers in a region with the most up-to-date information on toxicity, poisoning, and overdose.

References — Chapter 24

American Association of Poison Control Centers. "Criteria for Designation as a Regional Poison Control Center." *Vet. Hum. Toxicol.* 27:246-250, 1985.

C. S. Conner, A. S. Watanabe, and B. H. Rumack, "Drug Information — The Problems and Some Solutions." *Drug Intell. Clin. Phar.* 13:86-93, 1979

M. S. McIntyre, and C. R. Angle, "Regional Poison Control Centers Improve Patient Care." *N. Engl. J. Med.* 308:219, 1983.

R. Sagotsky, W. A. Gouveia, and F. H. Lovejoy, "Evaluation of the Effectiveness of a Poison Information Center." *Clin. Toxicol.* 11:581-586, 1977.

A. R. Temple, "Poison Control Centers: Prospects and Capabilities." *Ann. Rev. Pharmacol. Toxicol.* 17:215-222, 1977.

J. C. Veltri, "Toxicology Information Resources for Poison Control Centers." *Clin. Toxicol.* 12:335-356, 1978.

J. M. Waldman, H. C. Mofensen, and J. Greensher, "Evaluating the Functioning of a Poison Control Center." *Clinical Pediatr.* 15:75-80, 1976.

BIBLIOGRAPHY

Arena, Jay M. *Poisoning-Toxicology-Symptoms-Treatments*, 4th ed. Springfield, IL: Charles C. Thomas, Publisher, 1979.

Brown, John H. *Toxicology and Pharmacology of Venoms from Poisonous Snakes*. Springfield, IL: Charles C. Thomas, Publisher, 1973.

Czajka, Peter A., and Duffy, James P. *Poisoning Emergencies (A Guide for Emergency Medical Personnel)*. St. Louis: C. V. Mosby, 1980.

Dreisbach, Robert H. *Handbook of Poisonings*, 10th ed. Los Altos, CA: Lange Medical Publications, 1983.

Gilman, Alfred Goodman. *The Pharmacological Basis of Therapeutics*, 7th ed. New York: Macmillan, 1985.

Goldfrank, Lewis R. *Toxicologic Emergencies — A Comprehensive Handbook in Problem Solving*, 3rd ed. Norwalk, CT: Appleton-Century-Crofts, Publisher, 1986.

Haddad, Lester M., and Winchester, James F. *Clinical Management of Poisoning and Drug Overdose*, Philadelphia: W.B. Saunders, Co., 1983.

Hanenson, Irwin B. *Quick Reference to Clinical Toxicology*. Philadelphia: J. B. Lippincott, 1980.

Hardin, James W., and Arena, Jay M. *Human Poisoning from Native and Cultivated Plants*, Durham, NC: Duke University Press, 1969.

Kingsbury, John M. *Poisonous Plants of the United States and Canada*. Englewood Cliffs, NJ: Prentice-Hall, 1964.

Lincoff, Gary, and Mitchell, D.H. *Toxic and Hallucinogenic Mushroom Poisonings*. New York: Van Nostrand Reinhold, 1977.

Russell, Findlay E. *Snake Venom Poisoning*. Philadelphia: J. B. Lippincott, 1980.

INDEX

The Catholic Health Association of the United States is the national service organization comprising Catholic hospitals and long term care facilities, their sponsoring organizations and systems, and other health and related agencies and services operated as Catholic. It is an ecclesial community participating in the mission of the Catholic Church through its members' ministry of healing. By providing leadership representative of its constituency, both within the Church and within the pluralistic society, CHA's programs of education, facilitation, and advocacy witness this ministry.

This document represents one more service of The Catholic Health Association of the United States, 4455 Woodson Road, St. Louis, MO 63134, 314-427-2500.